AF449211

Endoscopic Ultrasonography in Gastroenterology

Edited by

KEIICHI KAWAI, M.D.
Professor, Department of Preventive Medicine,
Kyoto Prefectural University of Medicine,
Kyoto, Japan

IGAKU-SHOIN   Tokyo·New York

Published and distributed by
IGAKU-SHOIN Ltd.
   5-24-3 Hongo, Bunkyo-ku, Tokyo
IGAKU-SHOIN Medical Publishers, Inc.
   1140 Avenue of the Americas, New York, N.Y. 10036

Library of Congress Cataloging-in-Publication Data

Endoscopic ultrasonography in gastroenterology.

   Includes bibliographies and index.
   1. Endoscopic ultrasonography.   2. Gastrointestinal
system—Diseases—Diagnosis.   3. Gastrointestinal
system—Ultrasonic imaging.   I. Kawai, Keiichi,
1932-   . [DNLM: 1. Endoscopy.   2. Gastrointestinal
Diseases—diagnosis.   3. Ultrasonic Diagnosis.
WI 141 E567]
RC804.E59E63   1988   616.3'307543   88-8429

ISBN 0-89640-151-0 (New York)
ISBN 4-260-14151-1 (Tokyo)

Printed and bound in Japan

Preface

The field of endoscopic ultrasonography (EUS) as a new technique was established by several international researchers. The first international workshop on EUS was held in Stockholm in 1982. At the same time the first cooperative work was directed by Prof. M. Classen and myself. Efforts aimed at opening up this new field were made, since we felt that the information should not be preserved among only researchers. Since 1982, four international workshops have been held and the results have been released in special issues of the *Scandinavian Journal of Gastroenterology* and *Endoscopy* in West Germany. All of the achievements accomplished so far are compiled in this monograph. This compilation reflects the advanced techniques and their place in the forefront of considerable competition.

With the help of ultrasonography, endoscopic diagnosis has made tertiary diagnosis possible. Most importantly, however, is the efficacy of the method, which has been brought to patients. It is hoped that this new modality will be evaluated in terms of results in advanced medical treatments, as well as its technological developments.

Keiichi Kawai, M.D.
Kyoto, July 1988

Contributors

Tsuyoshi Aibe, M.D.
The First Department of Internal Medicine, Yamaguchi University School of Medicine, Ube, Yamaguchi, Japan

Kazuo Baba, B.E.
Director, Baba Medical Engineering Laboratory, Hachioji, Tokyo, Japan

Luigi Barbara, M.D.
Professor and Director, Academic Department of Medicine and Gastroenterology, University of Bologna, Policlinico S. Orsola, Bologna, Italy

Luigi Bolondi, M.D.
Academic Department of Medicine and Gastroenterology, University of Bologna, Policlinico S. Orsola, Bologna, Italy

Giancarlo Caletti, M.D.
Academic Department of Medicine and Gastroenterology, University of Bologna, Policlinico S. Orsola, Bologna, Italy

Eisai Cho, M.D.
Department of Gastroenterology, Kyoto Second Red Cross Hospital, Kyoto, Japan

Meinhard Classen, M.D.
Professor and Director, II. Medizinische Klinik und Poliklinik der Technischen Universität München, Klinikum rechts der Isar München, Federal Republic of Germany

Henryk Dancygier, M.D.
Associate Professor, Head of Ultrasound Section, II. Medizinische Klinik und Poliklinik der Technischen Universität München, Klinikum rechts der Isar, München, Federal Republic of Germany

Morimichi Fukuda, M.D.
Professor, Department of Ultrasound and Medical Electronics, Sapporo Medical College, Sapporo, Hokkaido, Japan

Yoshiki Hayashi, M.D.
Second Department of Internal Medicine, Nagoya University School of Medicine, Nagoya, Japan

Kazuo Inui, M.D.
Second Department of Internal Medicine, Nagoya University School of Medicine, Nagoya, Japan

Keiichi Kawai, M.D.
Professor, Department of Preventive Medicine, Kyoto Prefectural University of Medicine, Kyoto, Japan

Michael B. Kimmey, M.D.
Assistant Professor of Medicine and Director of
Therapeutic Endoscopy, Division of Gastroenter-
ology, Department of Medicine, University of
Washington, Seattle, Washington, U.S.A.

Eizo Kimoto, M.D.
Second Department of Internal Medicine,
Nagoya University School of Medicine, Nagoya,
Japan

Keisuke Kiyota, M.D.
Department of Gastroenterology, Kyoto Second
Red Cross Hospital, Kyoto, Japan

William R. Lees, F.R.C.R.
Consultant Radiologist, Radiology Department,
The Middlesex Hospital, London, United
Kingdom

Roy W. Martin, Ph.D.
Research Associate Professor, Department of
Anesthesiology and Center for Bioengeneering,
University of Washington, Seattle, Washington,
U.S.A.

Satoaki Mima, M.D.
Chief, Division of Hepatology, Hokkaido Kin-
ikyo Central Hospital, Sapporo, Hokkaido,
Japan

Keiichi Morita, M.D.
Second Department of Internal Medicine,
Nagoya University School of Medicine, Nagoya,
Japan

Hidekazu Mukai, M.D.
Department of Gastroenterology, Kyoto Second
Red Cross Hospital, Kyoto, Japan

Yasuo Naitoh, M.D.
Second Department of Internal Medicine,
Nagoya University School of Medicine, Nagoya,
Japan

Masatsugu Nakajima, M.D.
Director, Department of Gastroenterology,
Kyoto Second Red Cross Hospital, Kyoto,
Japan

Saburo Nakazawa, M.D.
Associate Professor, Second Department of
Internal Medicine, Nagoya University School
of Medicine, Nagoya, Japan

Tsuguhisa Sasai, B.E.
Endoscope Section, Product Development
Department, Endoscope Division, Olympus
Optical Co., Ltd., Hachioji, Tokyo, Japan

Fred E. Silverstein, M.D.
Professor of Medicine and Director of Gastro-
intestinal Endoscopy Service, Division of Gas-
troenterology, Department of Medicine,
University of Washington, Seattle, Washington,
U.S.A.

Tadayoshi Takemoto, M.D.
Professor and Chairman, The First Department
of Internal Medicine, Yamaguchi University
School of Medicine, Ube, Yamaguchi, Japan

T.L. Tio, M.D.
Division of Gastroenterology-Hepatology,
Academic Medical Center, University of Am-
sterdam, Amsterdam, The Netherlands

G.N.J. Tytgat, M.D., Ph.D.
Professor of Medicine and Gastroenterology,
Chief, Division of Gastroenterology-Hepatology,
Academic Medical Center, University of Am-
sterdam, Amsterdam, The Netherlands

Kenji Yamao, M.D.
Second Department of Internal Medicine,
Nagoya University School of Medicine, Nagoya,
Japan

Kenjiro Yasuda, M.D.
Department of Gastroenterology, Kyoto Second
Red Cross Hospital, Kyoto, Japan

Contents

1. **Instrumentation and Scanning Techniques** 1
Giancarlo Caletti, M.D., Luigi Bolondi, M.D., Luigi Barbara, M.D.

2. **Development of Ultrasonic Endoscope** 18
Tsuguhisa Sasai, B.E.

3. **Ultrasound Interaction with the Intestinal Wall: Esophagus, Stomach and Colon** 35
Michael B. Kimmey, M.D., Fred E. Silverstein, M.D., Roy W. Martin, Ph.D.

4. **Benign Lesions of the Gastrointestinal Tract** 44
Tsuyoshi Aibe, M.D., Tadayoshi Takemoto, M.D.

5. **Malignant Lesions of the Gastrointestinal Tract** 56
Kenjiro Yasuda, M.D., Masatsugu Nakajima, M.D., Keiichi Kawai, M.D.

6. **Pancreatic Cancer** 72
Henryk Dancygier, M.D., Meinhard Classen, M.D.

7. **Chronic Pancreatitis** 79
Saburo Nakazawa, M.D., Yoshiki Hayashi, M.D., Yasuo Naitoh, M.D., Eizo Kimoto, M.D., Kenji Yamao, M.D., Keiichi Morita, M.D., Kazuo Inui, M.D.

8. **Gallbladder Diseases** 87
Keiichi Morita, M.D., Saburo Nakazawa, M.D., Eizo Kimoto, M.D., Kenji Yamao, M.D., Yoshiki Hayashi, M.D.

9. **Diseases of the Biliary Tract and the Papilla of Vater** 96
Kenjiro Yasuda, M.D., Masatugu Nakajima, M.D., Keiichi Kawai, M.D.

10. **Evaluation of Resectability of Gastrointestinal Tumors** 106
T.L. Tio, M.D., G.N.J. Tytgat, M.D.

11. Laparoscopic Sonography in Differential Diagnosis of Liver Diseases
.... 119
Morimichi Fukuda, M.D., Satoaki Mima, M.D.

12. A. Future Perspectives of Endoscopic Ultrasound 132
William R. Lees, F.R.C.R.

B. Perspectives of Endoscopic Ultrasonography: A Review from a Medical Engineer's Viewpoint 138
Kazuo Baba, B.E.

13. Anatomical Aspects of Endoscopic Ultrasonography 140
Kenjiro Yasuda, M.D., Keisuke Kiyota, M.D., Hidekazu Mukai, M.D., Eisai Cho, M.D.

Index 159

1

Instrumentation and Scanning Techniques

Giancarlo Caletti, Luigi Bolondi and Luigi Barbara

In the last decade transcutaneous gray scale ultrasonography has progressed extensively in medical diagnosis. The heart, large vessels, and parenchymatous organs (such as the liver, pancreas, and kidneys) could now be visualized clearly with a safe, noninvasive and repeatable technique. However, certain organs could not be explored well because of bones and intestinal gas interference. Also, fat deteriorated the quality of transabdominal ultrasonic images. Intraluminal scanning has been considered to overcome these situations and to obtain a close scanning of intraabdominal structures. Because of this proximity, deep penetration of the ultrasonic beam is not necessary, which allows higher sonographic frequencies with greater resolution.

Wild and Reid in 1957 (19) first attempted blind intraluminal scanning of the rectum; since then, internal transducers are used routinely for prostate (rectal probes; 18) and bladder examination (transurethral transducers; 12). A transesophageal transducer has been proposed for M-mode cardiac exploration by Frazin and co-workers (9), and more recently also for bidimensional echocardiography (11). Intraluminal scanning of the upper abdomen, however, was delayed considerably because of the inability to introduce a scanning head safely into the stomach or duodenum through the esophagus, since these instruments did not provide endoscopic visualization.

Recently an ultrasonic gastrofiberscope has become available for clinical survey; preliminary results have been reported by Di Magno et al. (6–8). This instrument comprises a linear-array ultrasound system combined with an end-viewing endoscope. Several other systems have been built with different arrays combined with fiberscopes. The scopes can be end-, side-, and oblique-viewing. The ultrasonic apparatus can be linear arrays or mechanical or electronic sector scanning, with frequencies from 2.5 to 10 MHz. The depth of exploration can vary from 5 to 15 cm.

Initially, researchers' attention was dedicated primarily to obtaining a better view of the internal organs, especially those more difficult to explore by conventional ultrasonography: the heart, pancreas, and common bile duct (15). Increasing attention is now being paid to studies of the intestinal wall itself (3, 4, 7, 16, 17), and there is no competing technique for this application.

INSTRUMENTS

SECTOR SCANNING

The Olympus Company of Tokyo has the greatest experience in researching and developing sector scanners. Three prototypes of ultrasonic gastrofiberscopes have been provided for clinical evaluation.

The first prototype, a very preliminary one, was made only in few models. The ultrasonic probe was incorporated into the tip of a side-viewing gastrofiberscope (Olympus GF-B3). The images were scanned within a 90° sector in the direction of observation. The ultrasonic probe was covered by a balloon containing olive oil as a transmitting medium. The reflector rotated 4 to 8 times per second. The frequency was of 5 MHz with a depth of 3 cm. The length of the rigid tip was 8 cm (!) and its diameter 1.3 cm (14).

The second prototype of the device, which became available a year or so later, was markedly improved in its construction and in the scanning mechanism of the scope. Major changes were a small transducer with an increased frequency and direct rotation of the transducer connected to the flexible shaft. The scanning angle increased to 180° and the rigid part of the scope was shortened to 4.5 cm; the scanning head could now be introduced safely into the gastric as well as the duodenal lumen. However, these two prototypes could not freeze images.

In the Olympus prototype III, the ultrasonic probe is incorporated into the tip of a front oblique-viewing endoscope with a viewing direction of 70° forward-oblique and an angle of view field of 80°. The mechanically-rotating ultrasonic transducer produces a sector scan display of 180° or 90°. The frequency of the transducer is 7.5 MHz, and there are 10 display frames per second. The maximum displayable depth is 10 cm, focused at 3.5 cm. The rigid tip of the instrument is 4.5 cm long and 1.3 cm wide. This prototype can freeze images.

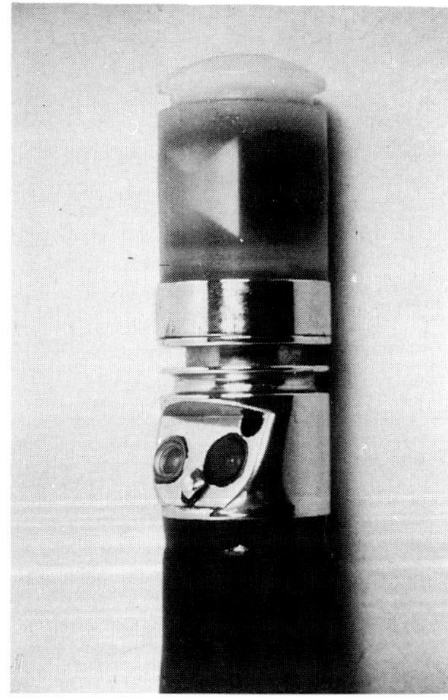

Fig. 1-1. Details of the tip of the sector scan Olympus GF-UM2.

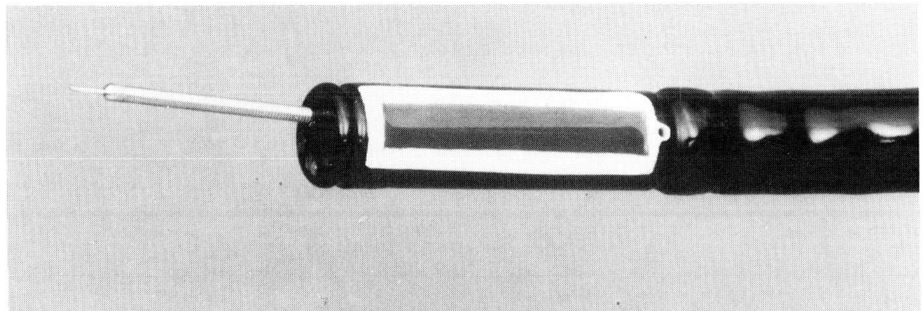

Fig. 1-2. Distal end of the linear-array Machida EPB-503 BL.

Prototype IV, also made by the Olympus Company, is GF-UM2/EU-M2 (Fig. 1-1; see Figs. 2-12 through 2-14). The detailed specifications of this instrument are shown in Table 2-2. Main improvements in this model are a shorter tip portion of the scope (3 mm less), a major flexibility of the shaft, a silent scanning, and the possibility of connecting instruments with different frequencies via different transducers. The focal distance is now 30 mm instead of 35 mm. Scanning is still mechanical, but the image display is digital rather than analogical. There is no biopsy channel in this scope, although this does not seem to be important. The ultrasonic unit has an angle of vision of 360° or 180° for a better orientation in the internal structures. The diagnostic field can be selected from 6, 9, 12, or 18 cm. Computer facilities are now available on the control panel.

LINEAR ARRAY

The most recent linear-array instrument available is the Machida EPB-503 BL (Fig. 1-2). The ultrasonic probe consists of a 5-MHz, 32-element linear array. The rigid tip is 45 mm long and 12 mm wide. This model has a channel for biopsy forceps or laser irradiation. The display unit (Toshiba SAL-35A or SAL-50A) produces an image 3 cm wide and 10 cm deep. A 7.5-MHz instrument can be used also, but without forceps channel (Machida EPB-703 FL).

EXAMINATION TECHNIQUE WITH A SECTOR SCAN ULTRASONIC ENDOSCOPE

We recommend that a complete upper gastrointestinal (GI) endoscopy be performed before an ultrasonographic examination. This examination will locate any lesion of the gastrointestinal wall necessitating an ultrasonic scan. Photos, brush cytology, and forceps biopsies must be done during the first investigation; in this way a good positioning of the ultrasonic scope will be easier, quicker, and more precise. In endoscopic scanning of extraluminal structures, a previous upper GI endoscopy is useful to recognize extrinsic compressions or to facilitate the progression of the ultrasonic shaft.

Endoscopic ultrasonography (EUS) is a long and heavy procedure for the patient. Therefore, we suggest that only one tract (esophagus, stomach, or duodenum) be investigated with a precise target.

After anesthetizing the throat with tetracaine (tablets) and administering intravenous Diazepam (5–10 mg) and Pentazocyne (15–30 mg), the patient is placed in the left lateral posi-

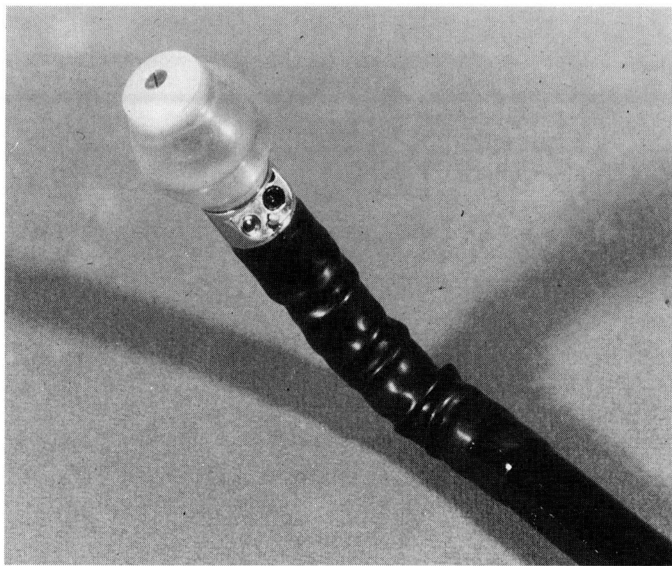

Fig. 1-3. Distal end of the sector scan Olympus GF-UM2 covered by the water-filled balloon.

tion and the instrument is advanced into the esophagus or stomach, and into the descending duodenum, if necessary.

EUS can be performed three ways: 1) by direct apposition of the transducer on the gastrointestinal mucosa; 2) with a small water-filled balloon covering the ultrasonic probe (Fig. 1-3); or 3) with a direct instillation of deaerated water (400–600 ml). The liquid for the balloon and for the stomach is injected with a syringe through a special channel of the fiberscope.

Direct apposition of the transducer on the gastrointestinal mucosa requires all air in the gut to be aspirated. The probe therefore is in close proximity to the intestinal wall and ultrasounds can penetrate without interference. This method is used mainly to explore large and easily identifiable extraluminal structures.

A water-filled balloon covering the ultrasonic probe allows separation of the probe from the intestinal wall, which in turn allows a good focus of the wall and the adjacent organs.

Direct instillation of deaerated water allows a good distention of the stomach (and/or duodenum); good visualization of the gastric (duodenal) wall structure is enhanced through the water. Moreover, small structures outside the wall that are difficult to localize are well studied with this technique. To facilitate the complete distention and to avoid peristaltic contraction, 20 to 40 mg Hyoscine N-butylbromide, or 1 mg Glucagon, are administered intravenously.

Various structures can be examined by more than one method, but the most appropriate technique for each organ is described in Table 1-1. Various organs can be visualized outside the different GI tracts, and are described in Tables 1-2 and 1-3.

Table 1-1. Method of choice for each structure exploration.

Direct apposition of the ultrasonic probe	Heart Aorta Mediastinum Spleen Gallbladder Right kidney Liver
Water-filled balloon	Esophageal wall Head of the pancreas Common bile duct
Instillation of water into the stomach or duodenum	Gastric wall Portal vessels Body and tail of the pancreas Duodenal wall Papilla of Vater

Table 1-2. Anatomical structures visualized from the esophagus and the stomach.

Esophagus	Anterior wall	Heart (4 and 5 chambers) Left atrium, mitral valve, left ventricle Coronary sinus
	Posterior wall	Aortic arch Descending aorta (cross-section)
Fundus of the stomach	Posterior lateral wall	Spleen Left kidney Tail of the pancreas
Body of the stomach	Posterior wall	Aorta (cross-section) Major branches of aorta Splenic vein (longitudinal section) Body of the pancreas
	Lesser curve	Liver (left lobe)

Table 1-3. Anatomical structures visualized from the antrum and from the duodenum.

Antrum	Posterior wall	Inferior vena cava Portal vein Body of the pancreas
	Anterior wall	Liver parenchyma
Duodenal bulb		Gallbladder Liver Portal vein Pancreatic head
Descending duodenum		Common bile duct Pancreatic head Superior mesenteric vein Inferior vena cava Gallbladder
Lowest part of Descending duodenum		Inferior vena cava Aorta Right kidney

EXAMINATION TECHNIQUE WITH THE LINEAR-ARRAY ULTRASONIC ENDOSCOPE

The linear-array ultrasonic endoscope is used most successfully with the direct apposition of the probe and water-filled techniques, depending on the examined organ (1, 13). (The balloon method is seldom employed with this scope.) Maneuverability and orientation are difficult with this instrument, because the optic and scanning parts are on different axes. Esophageal and extraesophageal structures are better and more easily studied than stomach or extragastric structures. For the same reason, scanning of small lesions may be time-consuming, owing to difficulties in localizing them (13). The special indications in using the linear-array scope still are not clear. Experts generally have used one or the other type of instrument, rather than both. Currently, the sector scanner has wider applications owing to its larger field of view.

RESULTS AND COMPLICATIONS

Swallowing of the instrument may be difficult, but accurate premedication can overcome this problem. In our experience, only 0.8% of patients could not swallow the shaft. Passage of the pylorus and descent into the second portion of the duodenum in normal patients was arduous with prototypes II and III; with model IV, our failure rate is only 15%. Complications owing to balloon rupture or water (from the stomach) aspiration into the airway have not been encountered (10).

SPECIAL PROBLEMS IN EXAMINATION

ESOPHAGUS

The esophagus can be explored ultrasonically by direct apposition of the transducer on the mucosa or with a water-filled balloon. In both cases, air must be accurately aspirated before beginning the examination. With the direct apposition of the transducer on the esophageal mucosa, structures outside this organ are well visualized, but the esophageal wall is not clearly identified. With the water-filled balloon, the wall structure is fairly well observed. Characteristic layers (as in the stomach) are identified if the balloon is not inflated excessively; otherwise, the wall is flattened. Large esophageal varices are visualized with the first method, but small varices and intramural and periesophageal vessels are better studied with the water-filled balloon (5). For these reasons we suggest exploring the esophagus starting from the cardia and going back slowly, always with the balloon on, which can be filled when necessary.

Within the esophagus there are two scanning obstacles, one related to the wall, the other related to the extraluminal organs. Fresh resection specimens of the esophageal wall show six echographic layers. They can be seen with the GF-UM2/EU-M2 when the probe is at least 2 cm from the wall (Fig. 1-4). When the probe is nearer than 2 cm to the tissue, only three layers are recognizable. In vivo, only three layers are seen (Figs. 1-5, 1-6). This difference in visualization is probably caused by a focus problem of the 7.5 MHz probe. Anatomical correspondence of these layers will be discussed later in this chapter.

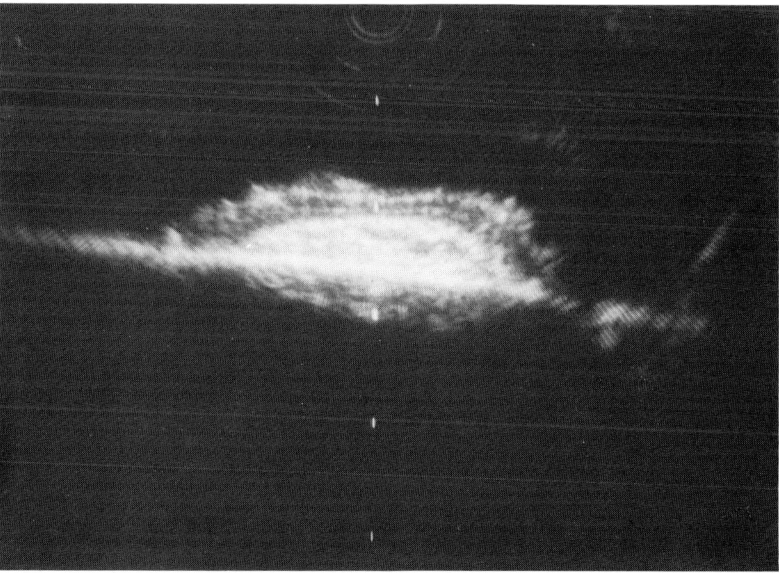

Fig. 1-4. In vitro under-water examination of the esophageal wall with the 7.5 MHz sector scan Olympus GF-UM2 at correct distance.

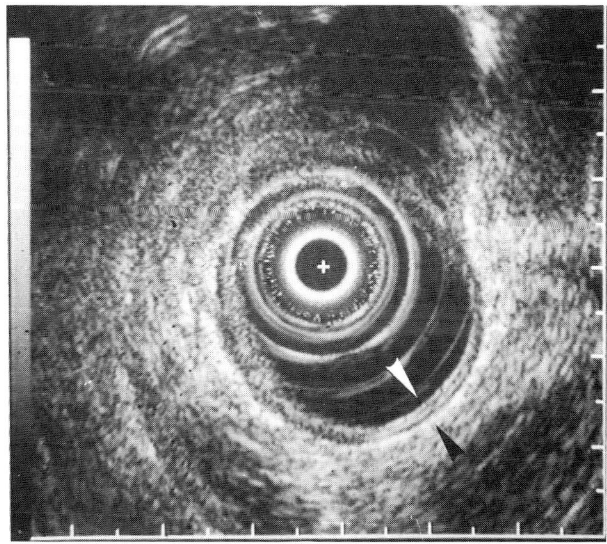

Fig. 1-5. In vivo examination of the esophageal wall with the 10 MHz sector scan Olympus GF-UM2 with the balloon technique. When the probe is 2 cm away from the wall, five layers are recognizable (see arrows). Under that distance only three layers are displayed.

When a lesion of the wall is scanned, its localization must be delimited by a previous conventional upper GI endoscopy, because only limited endoscopic visualization is available with the ultrasonic scope in the esophagus. Thus, the shaft can be advanced only with the help of its distance markers. Scanning a lesion in the upper esophagus is difficult because of the blind progression in that region. Orientation and identification of extraesophageal organs

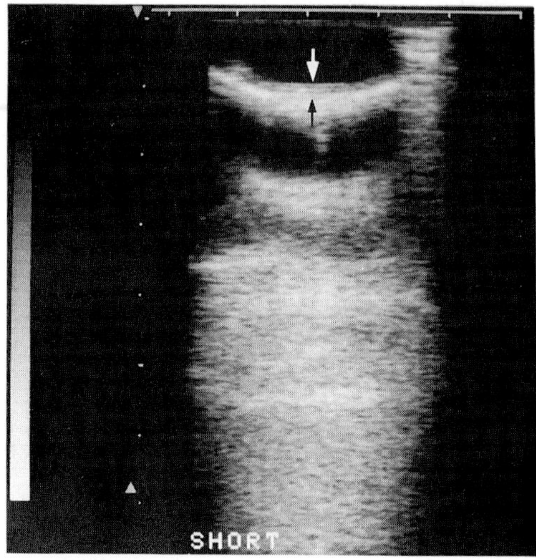

Fig. 1-6. In vivo examination of the esophageal wall with the linear array at 5 MHz. Machida EPB-503BL at correct distance.

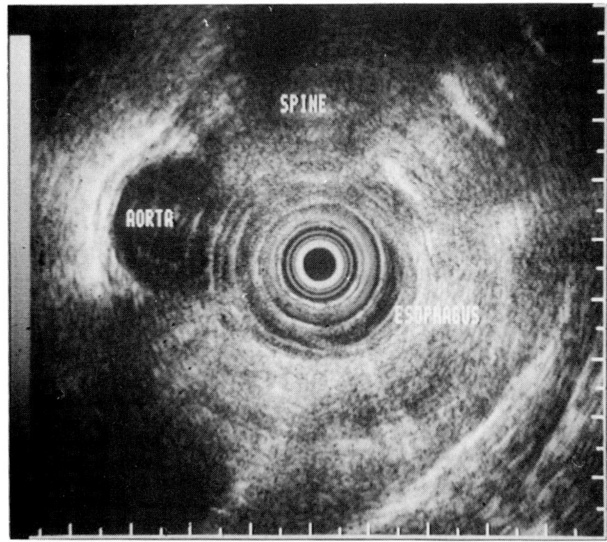

Fig. 1-7. Sector scan EUS in the esophagus.

is simple: there is no difficulty regarding scanning angle because the ultrasonic probe can move only up or down. Therefore, the scan is always transverse. The spine and aorta are always easily seen, and can often orient the observer in image interpretation (Fig. 1-7). Relationships between the esophagus and the aorta can be well studied; however, owing to air interference, the trachea corresponds poorly.

STOMACH

The stomach can be explored with all the three methods. With direct apposition of the transducer on the mucosa, structures outside the wall are explored (Table 1-1 and Fig. 1-8). With

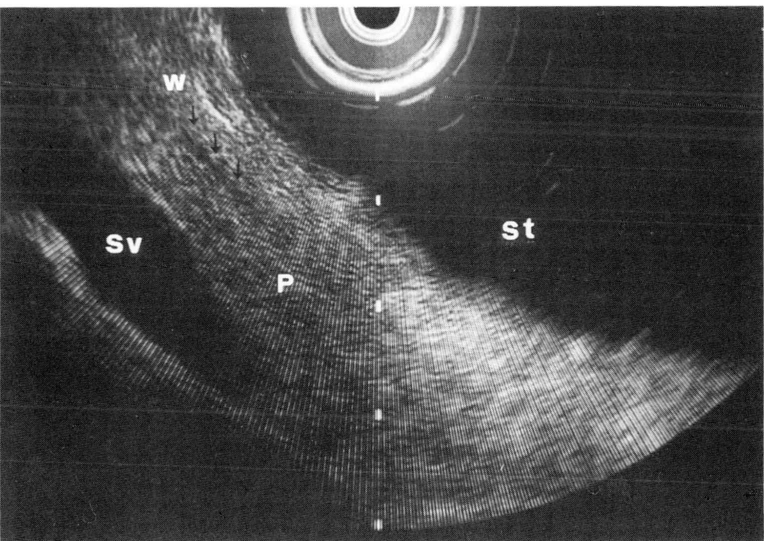

Fig. 1-8. Sector scan EUS of the pancreas. St = stomach; P = pancreas; W (arrows) = Wirsung's duct; Sv = splenic vein.

the water-filled balloon technique, extraluminal structures and the gastric wall are partially observed. Organs outside the gastric wall are too far from the focus and the gastric wall is not distended, so its characteristic layers are not clearly seen. For this reason we suggest that EUS exploration of the stomach be performed without the inflated balloon. With the last method, deaerated water is injected directly into the stomach through a special channel of the scope. Normally, 600 ml water will unfold the wall. When filled, complete exploration of the organ is achieved. For a complete ultrasonographic examination of the stomach we have standardized five positions.

Position 1
In postion 1 (Fig. 1-9), the tip of the instrument is in the antral region near the pylorus, lying on the great curve (GC) with the ultrasonic beam directed toward the lesser curve (LC). The screen displays a 360°/180° view of the antral wall. The anterior wall (AW) is on the left side of the image, the LC is on the bottom, and the posterior wall (PW) is on the right side (Fig. 1-10). The GC is partially visualized on the top.

Position 2
In position 2 (Fig. 1-11), the scope is shortly withdrawn and tip is bent upward until the body of the stomach appears. The ultrasonographic image on the screen shows the antrum as described for position 1; below it is the body. Its LC is strictly adjacent to the antral LC, and this double wall image corresponds with the angle area. The GC of the body appears on the lower bottom (Figs. 1-12, 1-13). In this position with a 360° scan the antral GC at the top of the image is well visualized.

Position 3
In position 3 (Fig. 1-14), withdrawing the endoscope into the body just before the angle area produces a reverse visualization. The body is displayed in the upper part of the screen and the

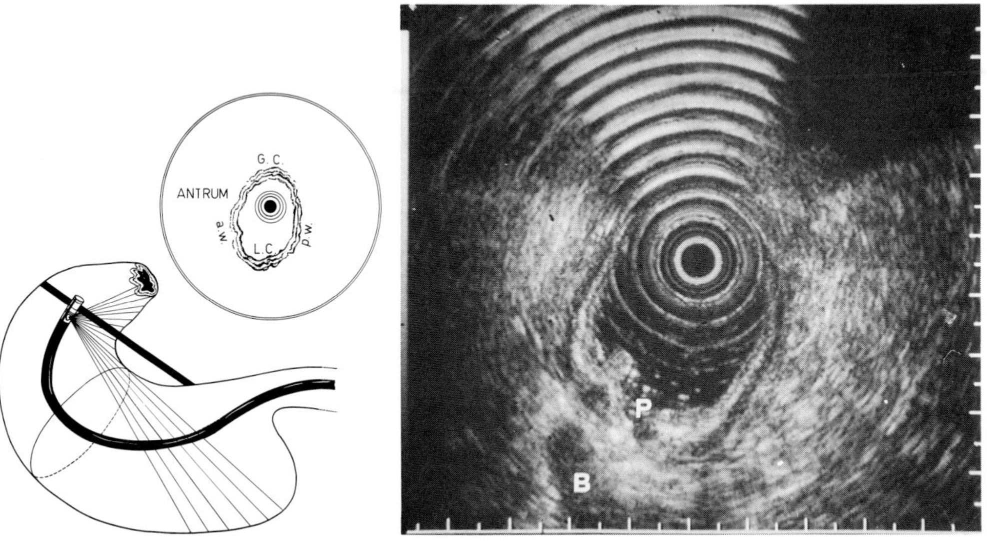

Fig. 1-9. **Fig. 1-10.**

Fig. 1-9.   Sector scan EUS of the stomach: first position.
Fig. 1-10.   In vivo image of Fig. 1-9.   P = pylorus; B = duodenal bulb.

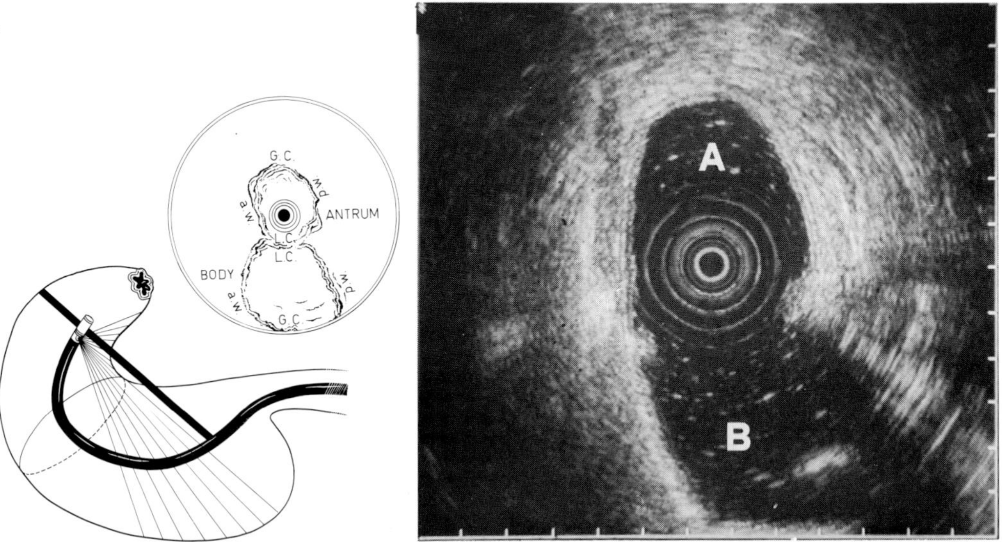

Fig. 1-11. **Fig. 1-12.**

Fig. 1-11.   Sector scan stomach examination in the second position.
Fig. 1-12.   In vivo image of Fig. 1-11.   360° examination.   A = antrum; B = body.

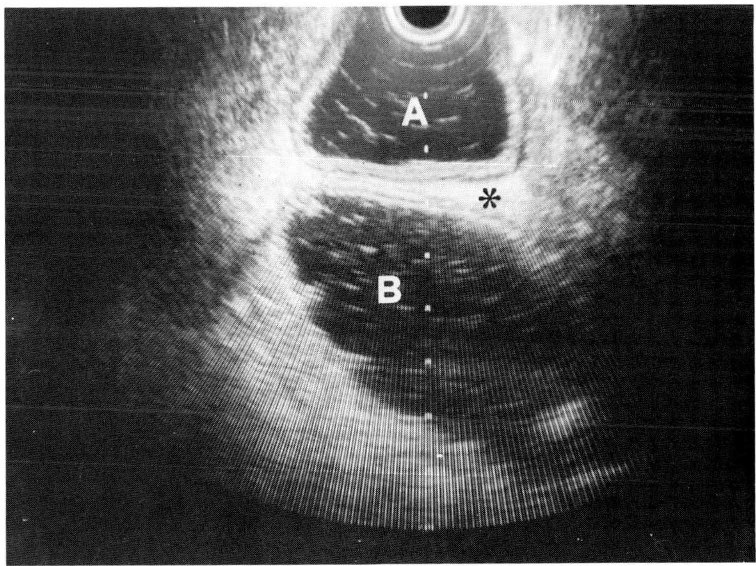

Fig. 1-13. In vivo image of Fig. 1-11. 180° examination. A = antrum; B = body; * = angle region.

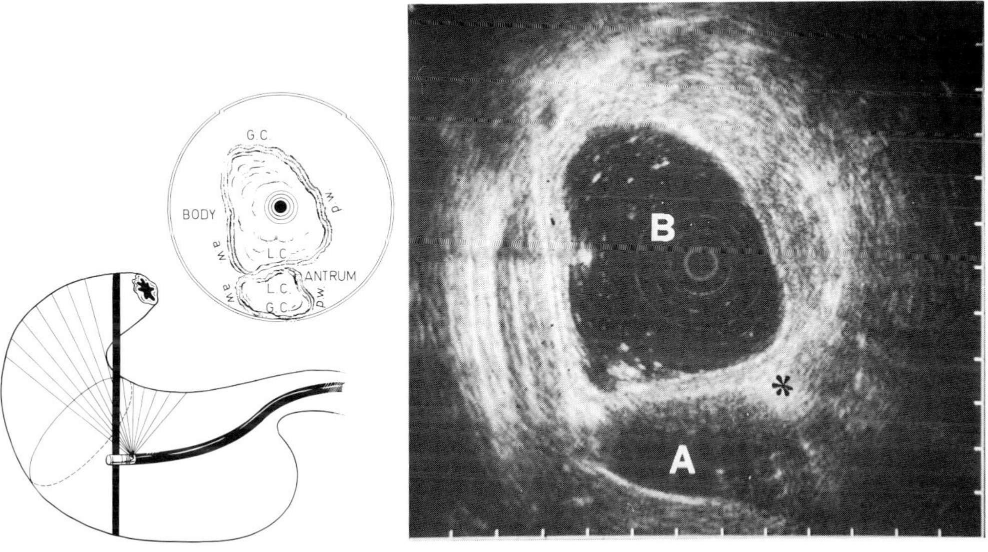

Fig. 1-14. **Fig. 1-15.**

Fig. 1-14. Sector scan stomach examination in third position.
Fig. 1-15. In vivo image of Fig. 1-14. 360° examination. A = antrum; B = body; * = angle region.

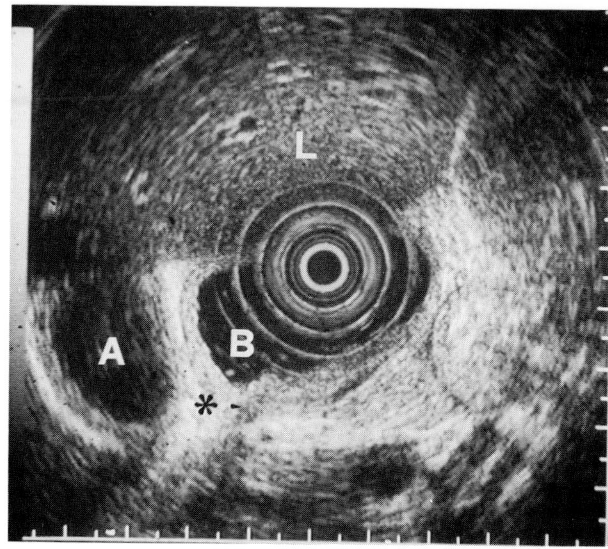

Fig. 1-16. The same as Fig. 1-15. L = liver.

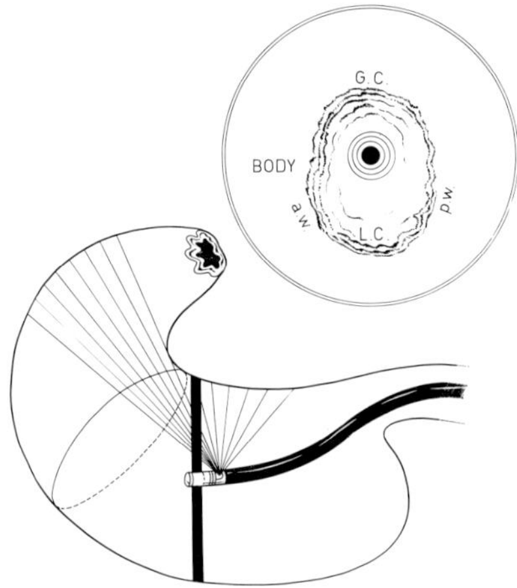

Fig. 1-17. Sector scan stomach examination in fourth position.

antrum in the lower. As previously described, the two sides of the LC appear strictly adjacent. The antral and body GC is so examined (Figs. 1-15, 1-16).

Position 4

In position 4 (Fig. 1-17), the endoscope is withdrawn further within the body facing the LC. With a 360° scan the whole body (LC, GC, AW, and PW) is displayed (Fig. 1-18).

Position 5

Position 5 (Fig. 1-19) allows the best visualization of the fundic area. The tip of the shaft is at the cardiac junction. The esophageal wall is visualized and at its side the fundus full of water is clearly pointed out (Fig. 1-20). When looking for a complete scan of the gastric wall a 360° or

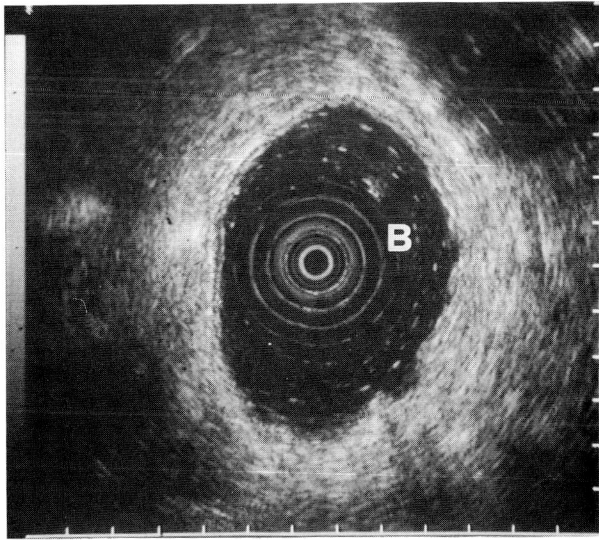

Fig. 1-18. In vivo image of the Fig. 1-17. 360° examination. B = body.

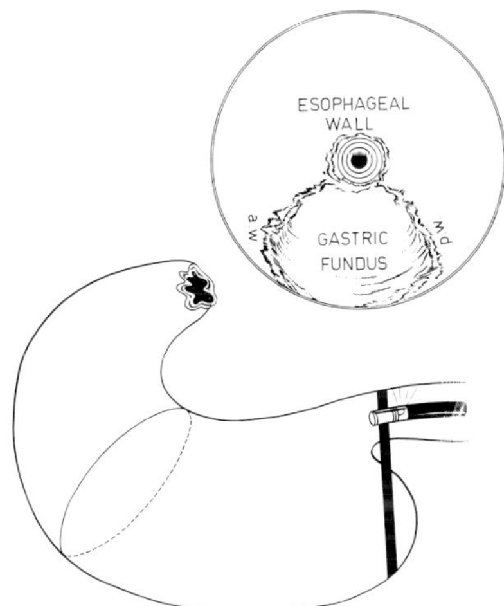

Fig. 1-19. Sector scan gastric examination in fifth position.

180° (up or down) display can be used. Total field display (360°) is useful for a complete and quick orientation, a 180° display (up or down) allows a magnification of the selected zone, fundamental in studying lesions situated distally on the screen. Only one region is nearly impossible to detect, despite a good and complete examination of the water-filled stomach: the upper part of the LC, just behind the cardia. This drawback occurs because of extreme proximity of the probe to the mucosa. Therefore, the probe must be focused at the right distance to obtain good images of the gastric wall layers.

Patients can be positioned differently from the left side when scanning a particular lesion. The right side provides good visualization of the antral region and the GC. The upward position allows one to study the AW, and the prone position is good to study the PW and pancreatic region. It is sometimes difficult to find and scan a small gastric lesion even though it

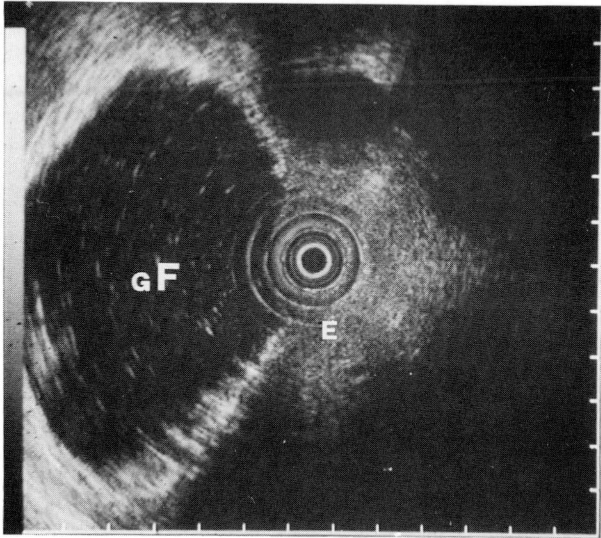

Fig. 1-20. In vivo image of Fig. 1-19. 360° display. gF = gastric fundus; E = esophageal wall.

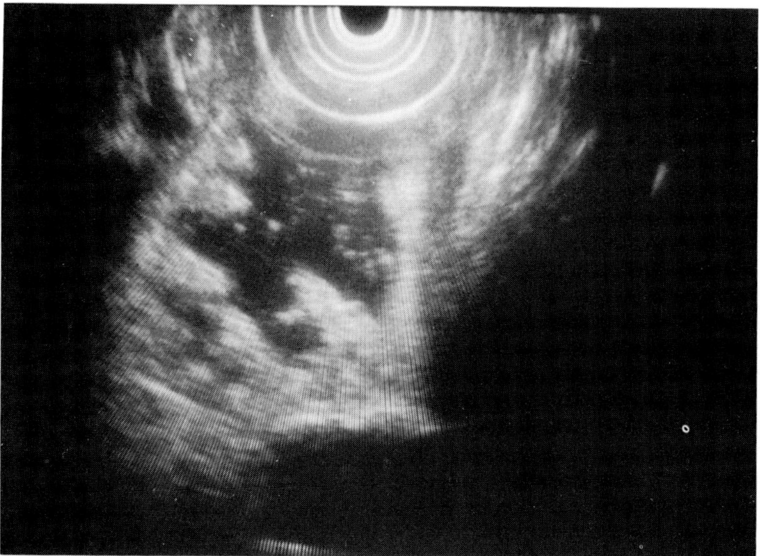

Fig. 1-21. Sector scan 180° duodenal examination.

is seen endoscopically because the optical tip and the ultrasonic probe are on different parallel planes.

DUODENUM

The duodenum can be explored with all three methods. With direct apposition of the transducer on the mucosa, only structures outside the wall are studied (Table 1-1). With the water-filled balloon method, extraluminal organs and the duodenal wall are partially observed. In both cases air must be aspirated accurately before beginning the examination. Unlike the esophagus and stomach, close contact of the ultrasonic probe with the duodenal wall is not achieved with these two methods, probably owing to the peculiar shape of the organ. In the left lateral position only the bulb and the internal part of the descending duodenum are carefully explored. To obtain a complete exploration of the second portion of the duodenum, it may be necessary to change the patient's position. For a study of the duodenal wall we recommend direct instillation of deaerated water: the descending duodenum is reached with the patient in the standard position; he is then turned in the right lateral position and 400 to 600 ml deaerated water is injected locally. The second portion of the duodenum, bulb, and sometimes the gastric antrum are well distended by the water and clearly visualized (Fig. 1-21). The examination is performed starting from the lowest part of the descending duodenum and slowly drawing back the instrument as far as the gastric antrum.

ECHOGRAPHIC PATTERN OF THE INTESTINAL WALL

As mentioned earlier, a major advantage of EUS is the ability to investigate the intestinal wall. The gastric wall comprises five layers (2, 3, 17) of different echogenicities (first innermost hyperechoic, second hypoechoic, third hyperechoic, fourth hypoechoic, and fifth hyperechoic) (Figs. 1-22, 1-23). Interpretations regarding the correspondence between these ultrasound features and real anatomical layers have been conflicting (12, 19). Our interpretation of the relationship of each echographic layer with a particular anatomical structure based on in vitro investigation (2), is that the first hyperechoic layer corresponds with the fluid/gastric mucosa interface; the second hypoechoic layer probably is produced as the ultrasound beam crosses the deep portion of the mucosa (including the muscularis mucosa, which is too thin to constitute a separate interface); the third hyperechoic layer corresponds with the submucosa and the submucosa/muscularis propria interface; the fourth hypoechoic layer is created as the ultrasound beam penetrates the muscularis propria, which is a relatively homogeneous structure; and the fifth layer corresponds mainly with the wall/fluid interface.

The thickness of these echographic layers changes in vivo according to the degree of distention and/or the functional state of the gastric wall. Different echographic layers usually are difficult to visualize in the esophagus, probably owing to difficulties in focusing the ultrasound beam on the wall, which is in direct contact with the transducer.

The esophageal normal wall presents six layers in vitro, provided the probe is a good distance from the mucosa, which is impossible to obtain in vivo. The fourth layer is separated by a thin hyperechoic layer in two hypoechoic layers, the middle hyperechoic layer interfaces between the circular and longitudinal proper muscle of the esophagus. Interpretation of other layers is the same as in the stomach.

In vivo only three layers normally are seen: the first hyperechoic corresponds to the mucosa-submucosa and submucosa-muscularis propria interface together; the second hypoechoic corresponds with the muscularis propria without a distinction between longitudinal and circular muscle; and the third hyperechoic is similar to the fifth layer of the stomach.

In the duodenum it is not possible to distinguish the five layers within the duodenal wall. The crescent-shaped folds show a homogeneous echopattern and only the muscular coat can be seen as a separate layer. The presence of the villi may account for the indistinguishable hyperechoic pattern of the mucosa and submucosa.

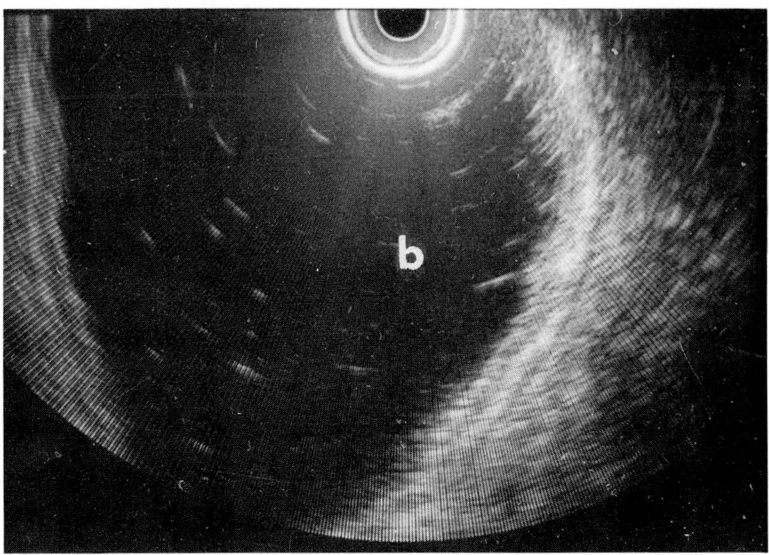

Fig. 1-22. Sector scan 180° stomach wall examination. b = body.

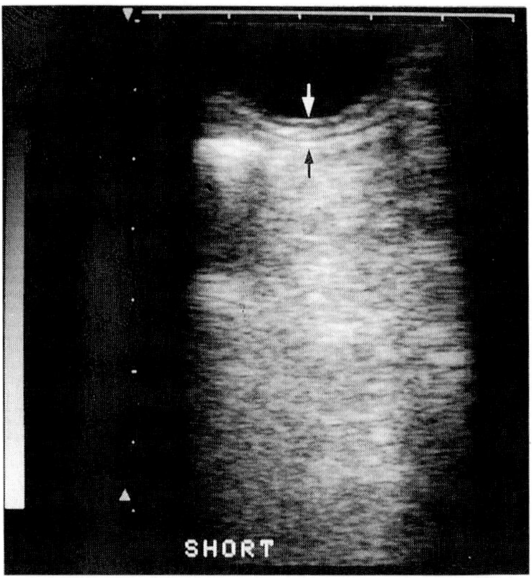

Fig. 1-23. Linear-array stomach wall examination.

FUTURE POSSIBILITIES AND IMPROVEMENTS

The role of EUS in the clinical diagnostic field, is continually expanding, with research and development of the instruments in progress. Thinner shafts and shorter tips are needed, and different frequencies for various investigations must be used. We are now testing the 10 MHz Olympus GF-UM2 for a more sophisticated investigation of the intestinal wall and we believe that it is necessary to advance in that direction to obtain new and unexpected results.

Aknowledgments

We thank Dr. T. Aibe from the Yamaguchi University School of Medicine, Japan, for photos and details concerning the linear-array ultrasonic endoscope, and Dr. Lorena Zani from our Department in Bologna University for help in translating, typing, and figure preparation, and for the enthusiasm in organizing this work.

References

1. Aibe T, Fuji T, Okita K, Takemoto T: A fundamental study of normal layer structure of the gastrointestinal wall visualized by endoscopic ultrasonography. Scand J Gastroenterol 21 (Suppl 123): 6-15, 1986.

2. Bolondi L, Caletti G, Casanova P, Villanacci V, Grigioni W, Labò G: Problems and variations in the interpretation of the ultrasound feature of the normal upper and lower GI tract wall. Scand J Gastroenterol 21 (Suppl 123): 16-26, 1986.

3. Caletti G, Bolondi L, Labò G: Anatomical aspects in ultrasonic endoscopy for the stomach. Scand J Gastroenterol 19 (Suppl 94): 34-42, 1984.

4. Caletti G, Bolondi L, Labò G: Ultrasonic endoscopy. The gastrointestinal wall. Scand J Gastroenterol 19 (Suppl 102): 5-8, 1984.

5. Caletti G, Bolondi L, Zani L, Brocchi E, Guizzardi G, Labò G: Detection of portal hypertension and esophageal varices by means of endoscopic ultrasonography. Scand J Gastroenterol 21 (Suppl 123): 74-77, 1986.

6. Di Magno EP, Buxton JL, Regan PT, Hattery RR, Wilson DA, Suarez JR, Green PS: Ultrasonic endoscopy. Lancet 1: 629-631, 1980.

7. Di Magno EP, Regan PT, Clain JE, James EM, Buxton JL: Human endoscopic ultrasonography. Gastroenterology 83: 824-829, 1982.

8. Di Magno EP, Silverstein FE, Giuliani D, Franklin D, Ohmori S: An improved ultrasonic endoscope: Preliminary canine experiments. Gastrointest Endosc 28: 129-130, 1982.

9. Frazin MJ, Talano JV, Stephanides L, Loeb MS, Kopel L, Gunmar RM: Esophageal echocardiography. Circulation 54: 102-108, 1976.

10. Fukuda M, Nakano Y, Saito K, Hirata K, Terada S, Urushizaki I: Endoscopic ultrasonography in diagnosis of pancreatic carcinoma. The use of a liquid-filled stomach method. Scand J Gastroenterol 19 (Suppl 94): 65-76, 1984.

11. Hisanaga K, Hisanaga A, Hibi N, Nishimuzaka K, Kambe T: High speed rotation scanner for transesophageal cross-sectional echocardiography. Am J Cardiol 46: 837-842, 1980.

12. Holm HH, Northved A: Transurethral ultrasonic scanner. J Urol 111: 238-241, 1974.

13. Rifkin MD, Gordon SJ: Sonoendoscopic evaluation of extraesophageal and extragastric abnormalities: A review. Scand J Gastroenterol 21 (Suppl 123): 68-73, 1986.

14. Strohm WD, Phillip J, Hagenmuller F, Classen M: Ultrasonic tomography by means of an ultrasonic fiberendoscope. Endoscopy 12: 241-244, 1980.

15. Strohm WD: Limits of conventional abdominal sonography and feature of endoscopic sonography. Scand J Gastroenterol 19 (Suppl 94): 7-12, 1982.

16. Strohm WD, Classen M: Endoskopisch-sonographische Diagnostik der Magenwand. Dtsch Med Wschr 108: 1425-1427, 1983.

17. Tanaka Y, Yasuda K, Aibe T, Fuji T, Kawai K: Anatomical and pathological aspects in ultrasonic endoscopy for GI tract. Scand J Gastroenterol 19 (Suppl 94): 43-50, 1984.

18. Watanabe H, Igari D, Tanahasi Y, Harada K, Saitoh M: Development and application of new equipment for transrectal ultrasonography. JCU 2: 91-98, 1974.

19. Wild JJ, Reid JM: In Kelly E (ed): Ultrasound in Biology and Medicine. American Institute of Biological Sciences, 1957, 30-45

2

Development of Ultrasonic Endoscope

Tsuguhisa Sasai

HISTORY AND DEVELOPMENT OF THE ULTRASONIC ENDOSCOPE

In 1950 the first successful pictures of the internal walls of the stomach were taken by blind use of a gastroscope. Since then, the fiberscope has been developed to the point where the internal organs can be seen with unaided vision. Today the fiberscope and video-image endoscope are the essential medical instruments for observing, photographing, diagnosing, and treating various organs, and their use is not restricted to the upper digestive tract. However, they have drawback in that it provides only optical images of organ surfaces; it cannot produce any information about what occurs underneath.

Ultrasonic tomography, on the other hand, has been developed to diagnose the organs located in the body cavity. The merit of this technology is its bloodless and noninvasive character. It is widely used as an important instrument in such fields as internal and respiratory medicine, obstetrics, gynecology, and urology. However, conventional ultrasonic tomography, in which ultrasonic waves are applied from outside the body, does not always produce good images of some organs because of the attenuation of ultrasonic waves by the gas that is present in the body cavity and tracts.

As a developer of medical instruments, we have for some time been contemplating an ultrasonic instrument that overcomes the drawbacks noted above. One idea concerned an endoscope that images organs by applying ultrasonic waves from inside the body cavity. In this way, good images can be obtained of the body tracts and diseased organs near by without having the waves attenuated by the abdominal wall or gas. Believing such an idea would contribute substantially to the advancement of medicine, we began to develop the ultrasonic endoscope.

SCANNING METHODS

Two major methods of scanning are used in an ultrasonic endoscope—mechanical scanning and electronic scanning (Fig. 2-1). The first method scans by the mechanical movement of a single piezoelectric transducer. Its typical application is the mechanical radial scanning method. The electronic method scans by electronically switching several tens of piezoelectric

18

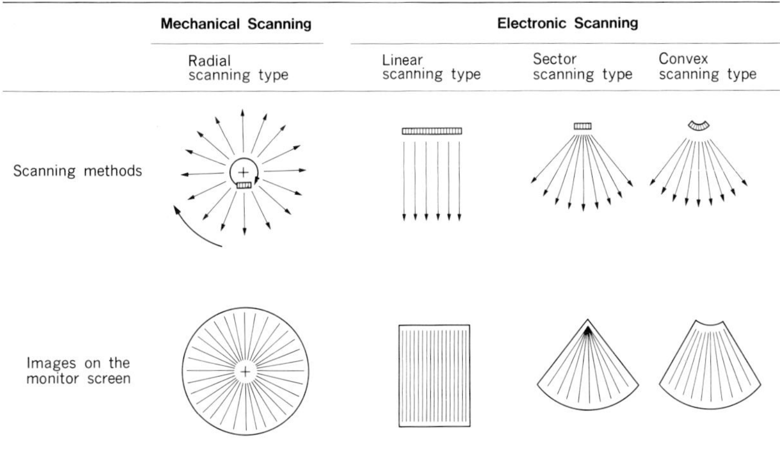

Fig. 2-1. Various types of scanning system.

transducers that are serially arranged and have a small rectangular parallelopiped shape. Typical applications are the linear, sector, and convex scanning methods.

The merits of mechanical radial scanning are its generation of high frequency ultrasonic waves by a thin piezoelectric transducer and its wider diagnostic field. The drawback is difficulty in achieving high scanning speeds because of the moving parts. The merits and drawbacks of the electronic scanning method are exactly opposite. The linear scanning method offers relative ease in handling regulation circuits and a uniform resolution when imaging organs located at short or long distances from the transducers. Its drawbacks are its long, rigid tip when equipped in the endoscope and difficulty in orienting the endoscope to the target organs, especially those located far from the transducers, because the diagnostic field is constant, narrow, and independent of the observation distance. The merit of the sector scanning method, in comparison with the linear scanning method, is that a wide, fan-shaped viewing field can be obtained using small piezoelectric transducers. The drawback is its complicated regulation circuits and narrow viewing field at short distances. The merits and drawbacks of the convex scanning method are somewhere between those of the linear and sector scanning methods.

DETAILS OF ULTRASONIC ENDOSCOPE DEVELOPMENT

We developed the ultrasonic endoscope based on the following fundamental criteria:
1. It should allow optical observation of the internal organs as well as diagnose the inside of the organs by the use of ultrasonic wave reflection.
2. It should give better resolution of organs than the conventional ultrasonic tomograph by using high frequency ultrasonic waves.
3. It should provide ultrasonic reflection images of the organs that cannot be imaged by conventional ultrasonic tomographs because of their anatomical location.

Based on the above criteria, we first considered possible target organs that can be effectively diagnosed using the ultrasonic endoscope (Table 2-1). We selected the pancreas, for

Table 2-1.   Target organs of intracavity ultrasonic diagnosis.

Scanning sites	Target organs for examination
Through the bronchus	Lymph nodes of the bronchus
Through the esophagus, stomach and duodenum	Heart Esophageal wall Gastric wall Pancreas Liver, gallbladder, bile ducts Kidney
Through the rectum	Rectal wall
Through the urethra	Prostate Urinary bladder
Through the vagina	Uterus
Through the abodominal cavity	Inside of the abdominal cavity

which the ultrasonic endoscope should be successfully applied in making a diagnosis. It is difficult to obtain good ultrasonic reflection images of the pancreas by conventional ultrasonic tomography because the gas present in the stomach and intestines decays the applied ultrasonic waves and because the pancreas is surrounded by the stomach, duodenum, transverse colon, and kidney.

On the other hand, the pancreas is suitably located next to the stomach and the duodenum. Therefore, if we could observe the pancreas from inside the body cavity using the ultrasonic endoscope, we expected to obtain good ultrasonic reflection images. Further, when ultrasonic waves are applied through the walls of the stomach or the duodenum, one need not worry about decay from the gas in the stomach or intestines.

Next, we chose the criteria for applying an ultrasonic endoscope in the diagnosis of the pancreas through the walls of the stomach and duodenum. The results are summarized as follows: (1) it should have the fundamental characteristics (observation, air and water supply, suction, and angling) provided by conventional endoscopes used for the upper GI tract, (2) it should be compact and provide high resolution images of the ultrasonic reflection of the organs, (3) it should be small enough to be inserted into the duodenum, and (4) it should not cause significant pain to the patient.

These four conditions provided the fundamental concepts of the ultrasonic endoscope, the so-called mechanoradial type in which a piezoelectric transducer is fixed at the tip of the endoscope having a side-viewing optical system for the upper GI tract and the scanning is made by a rotating mirror that reflects the ultrasonic waves. We did not use the electronic linear-type ultrasonic piezoelectric transducer, which was popular at that time, because we wanted (1) to make the length of the rigid tip of the endoscope as short as possible so it would be easy to insert into the duodenum for imaging the pancreas, and (2) to make easy orientation of the morbid focus of the pancreas in reference to surrounding organs.

Based on these fundamental considerations, we began the design of a trial ultrasonic endoscope in 1979.

FIRST TRIAL ULTRASONIC ENDOSCOPE

The aim of this development was to produce a trial instrument for evaluating the medical usefulness and technical possibility of the ultrasonic endoscope.

The appearance and specifications of the first trial ultrasonic endoscope are shown in Figs. 2-2, 2-3 and in Table 2-2.

Table 2-2. Specifications of various prototype instruments.

	1st Model	2nd Model	3rd Model (GF-UM1/EU-M1)	4th Model (GF-UM2/EU-M2)
Ultrasonic Endoscope:				
Frequency	5 MHz	7.5 MHz	—	—
Scanning method	radial scanning	—	—	—
	reflecting mirror method	rotating piezo-electric transducer	—	—
Scanning direction	vertical to insertion direction	—	—	—
Method of making contact	baloon method	—	—	—
		filling with deaerated water	—	—
External diameter of tip	13 mm	—	—	—
Length of rigid tip part	65 mm	45 mm	—	42 mm
Bending angle	up/down: 90°	130°	—	—
	right/left: 90°	—	—	—
Working length	1,100 mm	1,300 mm	—	—
Viewing direction	side-viewing	forward-oblique (70°)	—	—
Field of view	70°	80°	—	—
Channel	2 mm (opening for forceps not available)	—	—	—
Ultrasonographic Display:				
Presentation field	90°	180°	—	360°
Size (mm)	240 × 380 × 480	440 × 250 × 550	660 × 1,240 × 940	690 × 1,400 × 1,000
Weight	about 15 kg	about 30 kg	about 200 kg	about 110 kg
Photography	Pollaroid	—	Pollaroid, 35 mm	—
VTR recording	not available	—	available	—

—: same as the left column.

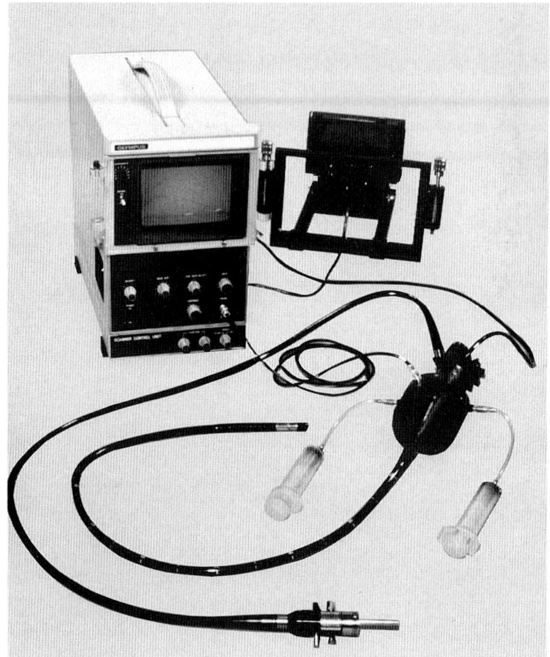

Fig. 2-2. General view of the first model.

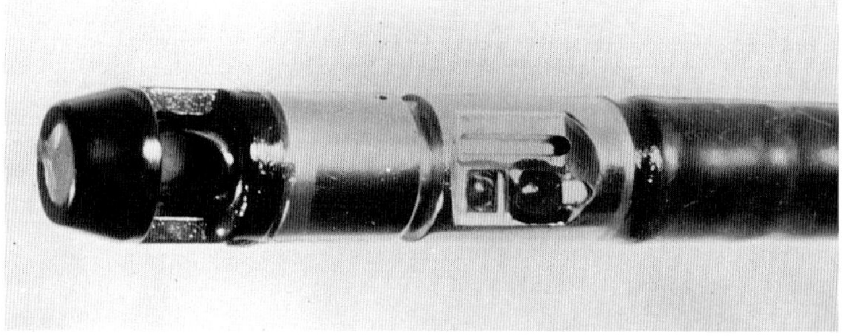

Fig. 2-3. Distal end of the first model.

Structure and characteristics

The structure and characteristics of the first trial ultrasonic endoscope are shown in Figs. 2-4 and 2-5.

We installed a single-plate piezoelectric transducer (PZT) with a 5-MHz ultrasonic wave frequency on a gastrofiberscope, GF-B$_3$, which had a side-viewing optical system. We used 5 MHz instead of 3.5 MHz that is popular in conventional ultrasonic tomographs because we expected high resolution images of the ultrasonic reflection since the trial instrument was free of the wave decay that results from gas in the belly wall and intestines.

Scanning was done by a rotating mirror that reflected the ultrasonic waves generated by the piezoelectric transducer, which was fixed at the tip of the endoscope. We used this system because we wanted a piezoelectric transducer with as large an internal diameter as possible. If we had used a rotating piezoelectric transducer instead, we would have had to transmit the

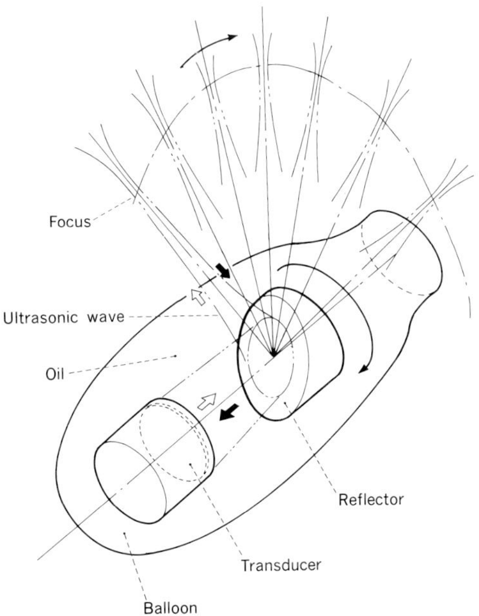

Fig. 2-4. Scanning mechanism of the first model.

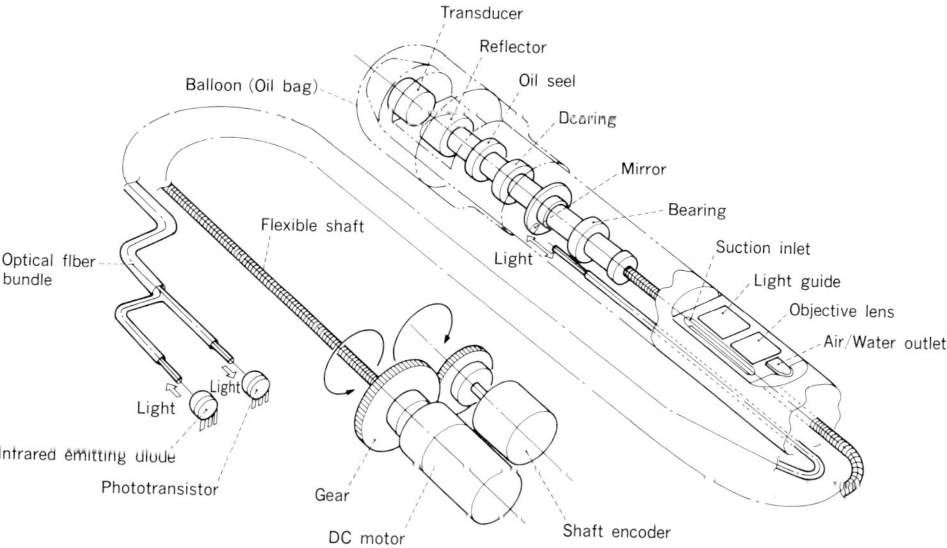

Fig. 2-5. Principle of the first model.

transducer's electric signals through rotatory electric contacts, making the system more complicated. By adopting this system, the rigid tip became as long as 65 mm, almost comparable to the tip of a gastrocamera. A motor in the sub-control section was connected to the reflecting mirror by a flexible shaft and supplied the rotation power. Detectors installed at the tip of the endoscope and in the sub-control section monitored the rotation speed of the reflecting mirror and the motor.

When we used this system, we covered the tip with a rubber balloon filled with olive oil in order to transmit the ultrasonic waves between the organ and the piezoelectric transducer. We favored the method of obtaining ultrasonic images of the pancreas by using a balloon in contact with the internal walls of the stomach and the duodenum, but we did not pursue the idea of filling the stomach with deaerated water.

Because of the application of the reflecting mirror system and its observational characteristics, the ultrasonic images were limited to the 90-degree cross-sectional area vertical to the central axis of the endoscope.

Problems encountered

Various problems were encountered with this first trial ultrasonic endoscope. Some major ones were related to the balloon, the flexible shaft, and the direction of image presentation.

We have improved the quality and shape of the balloon through trial and error. In some cases, bubbles formed in the balloon and could not be removed even when it was filled with olive oil. This made the pancreas diagnosis difficult because the bubbles appeared as white spots in the ultrasonic images. In some cases, the trial instrument performed very well during the tests, but in actual hospital practice the mirror stopped rotating because of friction with surrounding organs. Skillful technique by the physicians had to compensate for the defects in this first trial instrument.

The flexible shaft of the first instrument had difficulty in achieving a smooth rotation. As a result, the ultrasonographic images were severely deformed, an unacceptable condition for making a diagnosis of the organs. Later we improved the method of coiling, the quality of the shaft, and its heat treatment, and succeeded in getting a smooth rotation of the shaft.

To improve the direction of image presentation, we had to decide whether the top of the 90-degree, fan-shaped images (the piezoelectric transducer located at its center) should be displayed on the top or bottom of the monitor, and whether the cross-sectional images should be viewed from the tip of the ultrasonic endoscope or from the physician's side. We decided to follow the method used by CT scanner and by conventional ultrasonography. We presented the images of the piezoelectric transducer locus at the top of the screen, where they were viewed from the top of the piezoelectric transducer (i.e., the view is from the feet of the patient for cross sections of the upper GI tract).

We also had trouble with the instrument's durability. One example is the cracks that formed in the plastic fiber used to monitor the rotation of the reflecting mirror. This problem resulted in a cessation of the ultrasonic images, which meant that our instruments were often recalled from hospitals. We were kept busy troubleshooting these problems.

Results

This first trial instrument had operational problems such as: (1) heavy weight, (2) difficulty in filling and draining the olive oil from the balloon, (3) difficulty in insertion as far as the duodenum because of the large tip, and (4) severe pain experienced by patients even if it was successfully inserted into the duodenum. Another problem was that the images obtained by the instrument showed low resolution, although we had used the 5-MHz piezoelectric transducer, one grade above that used in conventional external ultrasonic tomographs. The viewing angle of the images obtained by this instrument was narrow (90 degrees), and it was difficult to orient the endoscope to the target pancreas or to pinpoint the pancreas locus.

Because of all these problems, the instrument was evaluated by physicians, who viewed it as comparable or inferior to conventional ultrasonic tomographs. The physicians were encouraging, suggesting that this instrument would become a useful medical tool when these problems were overcome.

SECOND TRIAL ULTRASONIC ENDOSCOPE

With the second trial instrument, we tried to solve the problems uncovered in the test operations of the first model. We especially sought to improve (1) the tip by making it more compact and easier to insert the scope into the duodenum, and (2) the resolution of ultrasonic reflection images by outstripping the conventional ultrasonic tomograph.

The appearance and specifications of the second trial ultrasonic endoscope are shown in Figs. 2-6 through 2-8 and Table 2-2.

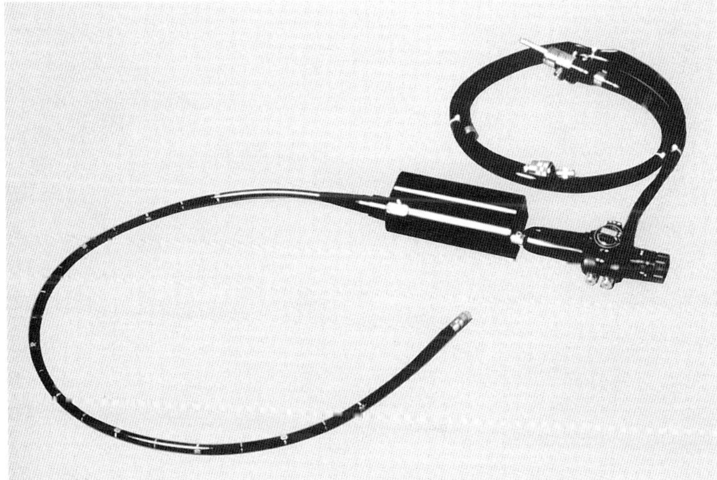

Fig. 2-6. General view of the second model.

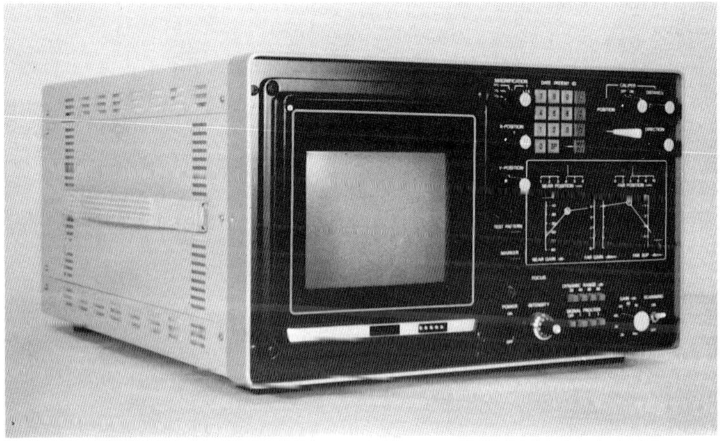

Fig. 2-7. General view of the second observing unit.

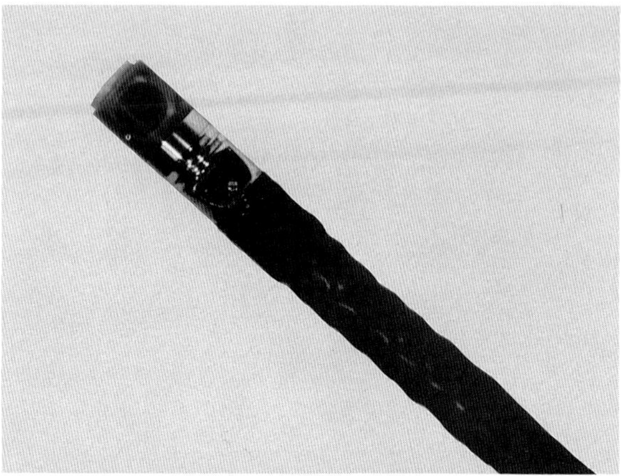

Fig. 2-8. Distal end of the second and third model.

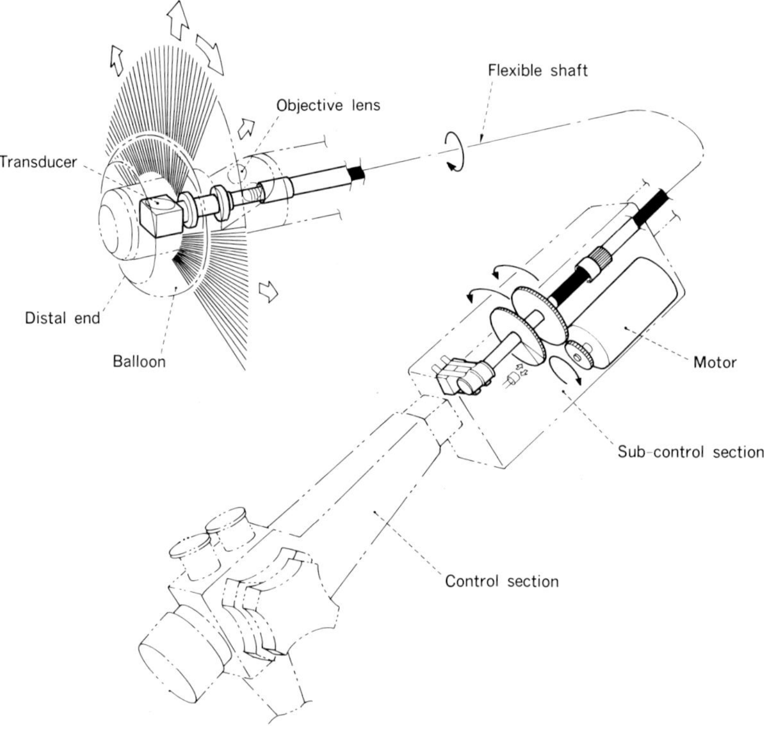

Fig. 2-9. Principle of the second and third model.

Structure and characteristics

The structure and characteristics of the second trial ultrasonic endoscope are shown in Fig. 2-9.

Because the first trial instrument proved difficult to insert into the duodenum and gave low resolution images of the organ, we abandoned the rotating mirror method of reflecting the ultrasonic waves. Instead, we decided to use a direct rotating method in which a rotating piezoelectric transducer was installed on the tip of an endoscope filled with oil.

This method allowed us to shorten the length of the rigid tip from 65 mm (the first trial) to 45 mm. We expected this to provide an easier insertion into the descending part of the duodenum. We also increased the ultrasonic wave frequency from 5 MHz, which had failed to give good resolution in the first trial endoscope, to 7.5 MHz. We also increased the viewing angle of the cross sections to 180 degrees by improving the observation system and making orientation of the instrument to the pancreas easier.

The optical viewing system was also changed to the foreoblique system. This allowed checking of the contact between the balloon and the cross-sectional part of the stomach and duodenum walls.

Problems encountered

Because we adopted the rotating piezoelectric transducer system, we had to transmit electric signals through rotary electric contacts, which complicated the structure of the endoscope. In particular, the electric cable, which rotated with the rotary piezoelectric transducer, had poor durability. It broke and stopped sending ultrasonic images about one month after delivery of the instruments to hospitals. During that period we were busy fixing broken wires during the day, and then working until late at night to design new methods to overcome the problem.

As expected, we did succeed in obtaining an easier insertion of the endoscope into the duodenum. But because the rotatory torque supplied by the motor to the piezoelectric transducer was not strong enough, the transducer frequently stopped rotating as a result of friction caused by the severe curving and bending angle of the flexible cable even if fully inserted into the duodenum. Some physicians, therefore, used the instrument not for diagnosis of the pancreas, but for the diagnosis of other organs to avoid inserting it into the duodenum.

Results

The shortening of the rigid tip made it possible to insert the instrument into the duodenum. However, this endoscope had poor durability in practical hospital use. The instrument was still incomplete considering the original purpose of applying it to the scanning of the pancreas through the wall of the duodeum.

On the other hand, several reports showed that the instrument could be effectively used in obtaining images not only of the pancreas but also of the stomach wall. This indicated usefulness in the diagnosis of the stomach. A new technique was proposed; good ultrasonic reflection images of the wall of the stomach could be obtained by filling it with deaerated water.

But this instrument was still incomplete because it gave unstable flickering images caused by the uneven rotation of the observation unit's motor. Images were recorded only by a non built-in Pollaroid camera or a 35-mm still camera, complicating the operation. It was also difficult to find good shutter opportunities to take pictures.

THIRD TRIAL ULTRASONIC ENDOSCOPE

We sought to improve the second trial instrument, specifically: (1) the quality of the ultrasonic reflection images so they could be effective for the diagnosis of the pancreas and stomach wall, (2) the stabilization of the transducer rotation after inserting it into the duodenum, and (3) the method of image recording.

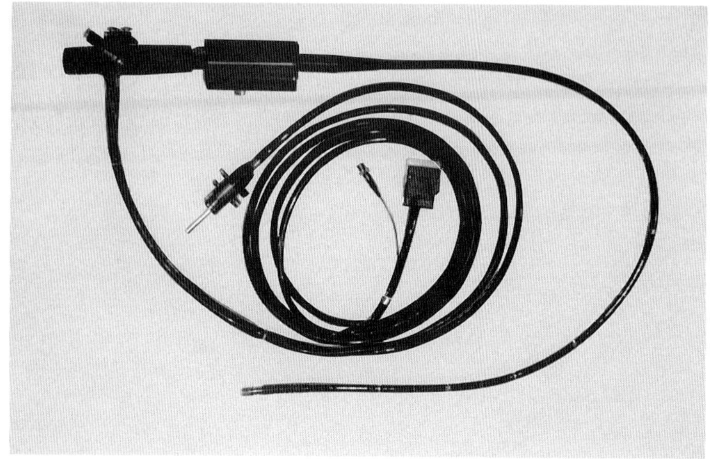

Fig. 2-10. General view of the third model ultrasonic endoscope (GF-UM1).

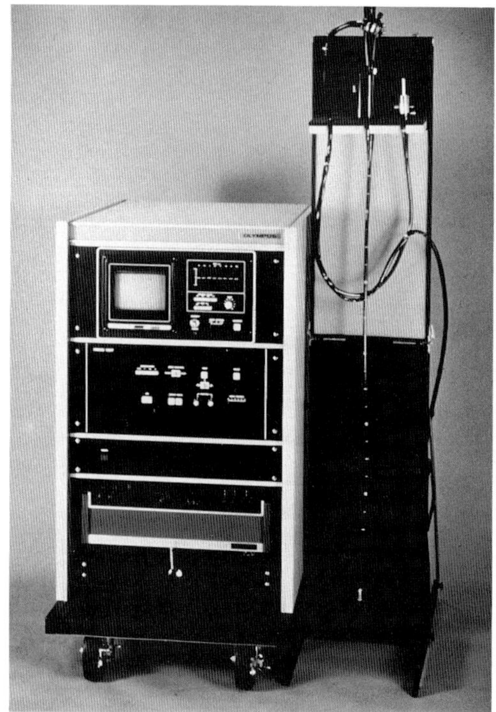

Fig. 2-11. General view of the third model system (GF-UM1 & EU-M1).

The appearance and specifications of the third trial ultrasonic endoscope are shown in Figs. 2-10, 2-11 and in Table 2-2.

Structure and characteristics

The structure and characteristics of the third trial ultrasonic endoscope are shown in Fig. 2-9.

The structure of the part to be inserted into the duodenum was the same as in the second trial instrument. However, we improved the sub-control section by installing a motor with high torque in order to solve the uneven rotation of the transducer that had plagued the second trial instrument. We made the sub-control section more compact for easier handling of the instrument. To get images with higher quality, we improved the quality of the piezoelectric transducer. We improved the observation unit by introducing a new circuit (DSC) and a new monitor (a high speed XY), expecting to get excellent resolution from the ultrasonic scanning section. An image inversion function was added to obtain cross-sectional images viewed from the direction of the operator. We expanded the practical viewing angle to 270 degrees by introducing an image rotation function. We also made possible VTR recording of images, feeling that it would help physicians in diagnoses if they could review recorded images of the target organs.

Difficulties encountered

Improvements and new functions were added to the observation unit. However, the poor durability problem of the second trial instrument was not solved. In particular, the electric cables suffered, and we could not find durable cable even after extensively testing various kinds of materials. The instrument also had other problems, such as: (1) leakage of oil in the flexible tube due to breakage of the tube covering the flexible shaft, (2) wear on the motor gears, and (3) abnormal noises produced by the mechanically rotating parts. Many changes were needed to improve its mechanical durability.

On the other hand, we were happy with the results of test experiments showing that the resolution and sensitivity of the instrument were much improved with the new piezoelectric transducer. We looked forward to the reports of physicians who were using the new instrument in hospital practice.

Results

The improved piezoelectric transducer and observation unit greatly aided the quality of the cross-sectional organ images obtained by the new ultrasonic endoscope. Many medical reports were made using the third instrument, such as the detection of small cancerous tumors in the pancreas, which has not been detectable by the conventional ultrasonic tomograph.

Use of the third trial ultrasonic endoscope in diagnosis of the stomach wall increased. Some research reports clearly revealed the five-layered structure of the stomach wall, indicating that the instrument could be applied to the diagnosis of stomach cancer by observing whether the submucosal layer was involved. This application had not been anticipated when we started development of the ultrasonic endoscope.

Since then, many reports have been made using the ultrasonic endoscope for diagnosing the wall of the stomach. This field of medicine seems open for major applications of the ultrasonic endoscope.

However, instrument durability was still not satisfactory. As well, the images recorded by the VTR could be visualized only with a special monitor system.

FOURTH TRIAL ULTRASONIC ENDOSCOPE

The aims of developing the fourth trial endoscope were: (1) durability improvement, (2) improvement of image quality to allow detection of small morbid targets in the pancreas and to clearly image the structure of the stomach wall, (3) easier assembling and disassembling of the instrument for the repair work required of the commercial product, and (4) fulfillment of a wide application range as a commercial product.

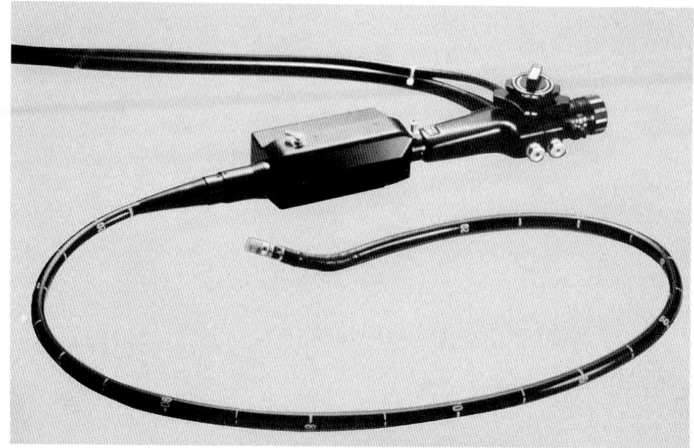

Fig. 2-12. General view of the fourth model ultrasonic endoscope (GF-UM2).

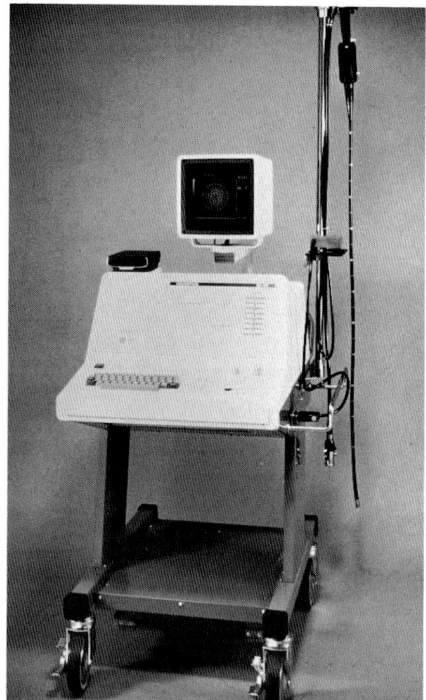

Fig. 2-13. General view of the fourth model system (GF-UM2 & EU-M2).

Considering all these factors, we planned to increase the functions of the instrument.

The appearance and specifications of the fourth trial ultrasonic endoscope are shown in Figs. 2-12, 2-13 and in Table 2-2.

Structure and characteristics

The structure and characteristics of the fourth trial ultrasonic endoscope are shown in Fig. 2-14.

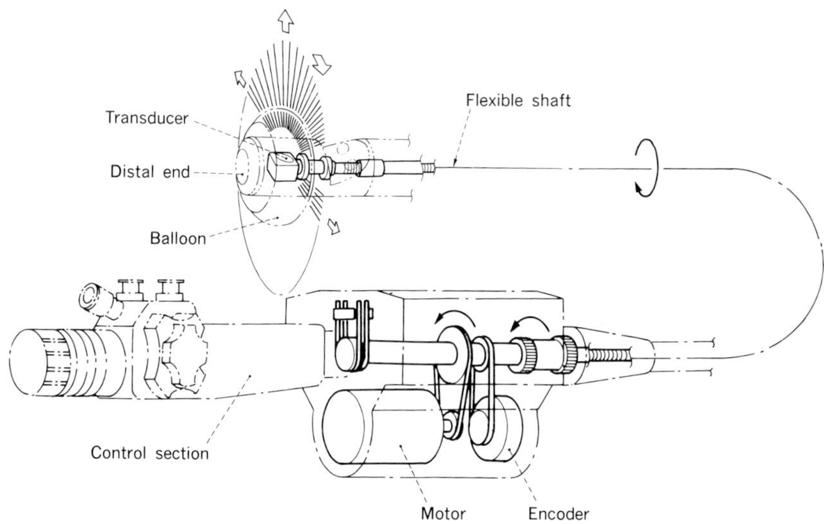

Fig. 2-14. Principle of the fourth model.

The fundamental structure of the fourth instrument was the same as the second and third. However, we tried to further easier insertion of the endoscope into the duodenum by shortening the rigid tip another 3 mm. We also tried to improve instrument durability, a major problem for a long time. We made several improvements to solve the problems of the electric cable being cut, the suction cock leaking, the oil leaking, image trembling, and wear on the gears. We also improved the observation unit and succeeded, for the first time, in widening the viewing angle to 360 degrees. We improved the electric circuit unit and made the recorded images reproducible on a conventional TV monitor. Functions for making distance and area calculations were also added.

Difficulties encountered
As noted, we worked hard to improve the durability of the instrument, which had been unacceptable in the earlier models. We spent busy days fixing the broken third trial instruments, testing the durability of the revised models, and then designing a new fourth instrument. However, we still felt that we could improve the instrument for commercial use, because the durability tests were encouraging.

The resolution of the scanned images was getting better and a 360-degree viewing angle had been achieved. We believed that the ultrasonic endoscope would become a valuable medical tool.

Results
Reports from physicians using the fourth trial instrument noted that it gave clear images of the organs, which could not been obtained with conventional ultrasonic tomographs. They also reported easier orientation of the endoscope than before because of the increased viewing angle of 360 degrees. The number of research reports using the new instrument grew larger. The target organs expanded from the pancreas and stomach wall to the walls of the esophagus, the rectum, and the bile duct. This tendency clearly indicated that we should study how far the ultrasonic endoscope could be applied for the diagnosis of various organs. The durability of the new instrument showed significant improvement, and it was stable enough to be inserted into the duodenum.

This fourth trial instrument was put on the market under the brand names of GF-UM2 and EU-M2. These instruments are now widely used by many physicians for the diagnosis of the stomach, pancreas, gallbladder and bile duct, and they are proving to be a powerful medical tool.

OTHER TRIAL ULTRASONIC ENDOSCOPES

In addition to the mechanoradial-type ultrasonic endoscope, we developed trial endoscopes based on electronic linear-type scanning using an electronic-linear piezoelectric transducer (Fig. 2-15) and an ultrasonic laparoscope for the body cavity based on electric-linear and the mechanoradial-type scanning (Fig. 2-16). We are trying to improve the performance of these ultrasonic endoscopes.

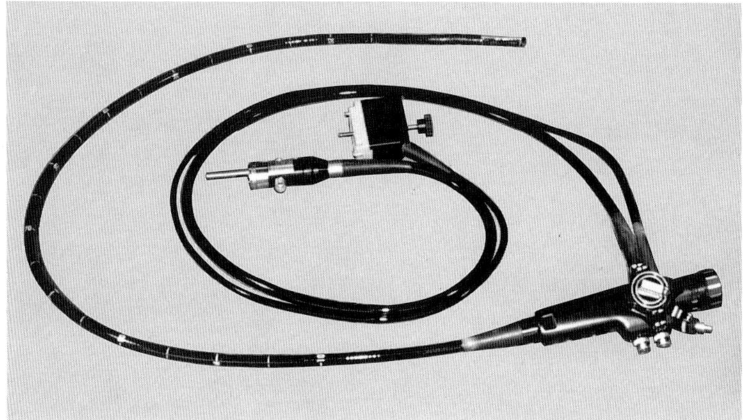

Fig. 2-15. General view of linear scan ultrasonic endoscope.

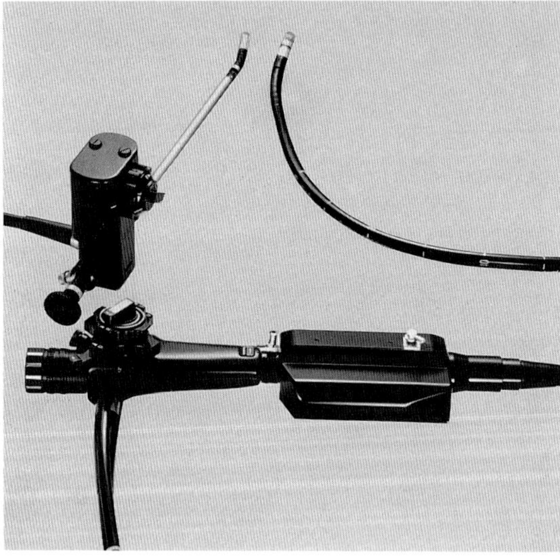

Fig. 2-16. General view of radial scan ultrasonic laparoscope and endoscope.

FUTURE PROSPECTS

The standard that physicians request for the performance of medical instruments is usually very high, even in the development stages. Requests for a higher standard for new instruments are a driving force that stimulates developers to improve their equipment. Such was the case with developing the ultrasonic endoscope. We greatly appreciate the guidance and suggestions of many physicians, without which the development of the present ultrasonic endoscope could not have been achieved.

Although the ultrasonic endoscope is just starting to flourish, there are already many requests for a more advanced version—the next generation of the machine (Table 2-3). Among these requests, an opening for forceps and the ability to switch the ultrasonic frequency have been achieved with the latest model, GF-UM3 and EU-M3. At present, a simple increase in frequency of the ultrasonic wave increases the loss of ultrasonic waves, making it impossible to reach long distances. However, this could be remedied with a pulse pressurization technique that would allow the wave to reach long distances. To make the instrument more compact, we hope to introduce an extremely small motor (such as an ultrasonic motor) in the tip of the endoscope to rotate the piezoelectric transducer. If we can remove the flexible shaft presently used for the transmission of the mechanical torque of the motor to the tip part, we can then make the insertion part of the scope slimmer and the sub-control section more compact. Possibly the piezoelectric transducer may become more compact while providing higher resolution with a transducer made of polymer.

An ultrasonic video endoscope equipped with solid imaging elements (CCD) in the tip has been already achieved, although there are still problems in that area, especially in making the CCD compact.

We can expect further development of image processing techniques in the near future. By various processings of the cross sectional ultrasonic images of organs (such as color presentation by coloring the images based on the strength of reflected ultrasonic echoes and stereo imaging by superimposing more than one cross-sectional image), we can obtain more data from the ultrasonic endoscope for the effective diagnosis of various organs.

Table 2-3. Requirements for improving ultrasonic endoscope.

Biopsy channel (EUS-guided biopsy)
Switching of ultrasonic frequencies
Compact form — Inserting unit (shorter and more compact tip, smaller diameter of inserting unit) — Sub-control section (compact and not heavy)
Instruments specific for various organs: — for the esophagus — for the lower GI tract — for examination of gastrointestinal wall — for the heart
Higher frequency
Equipment for color Doppler presentation (blood flow measurement)
Image processing: quasi-coloration, three-dimensional stereo imaging, other various processings
Ultrasonic video endoscope

Future diagnosis will be based not only on the images but also the examination of biopsy specimens taken from the organs with the aid of the ultrasonic endoscope.

It will take the absorption, utilization, and combination of new techniques to fulfill the requests for features to be incorporated into the commercial products. We believe we should further broaden the scope and improve the performance of the ultrasonic endoscope, thereby contributing to the development of medicine by manufacturing superior medical instruments. And we will continue to improve the ultrasonic endoscope so that it can be applied to the diagnosis of various organs.

3

Ultrasound Interaction with the Intestinal Wall: Esophagus, Stomach, and Colon

Michael B. Kimmey, Fred E. Silverstein, and Roy W. Martin

Diseases of the gastrointestinal wall can be difficult to diagnose when using traditional endoscopic and nonendoscopic techniques. Cross-sectional imaging of the gut, including percutaneous ultrasound, computed tomography, and magnetic resonance imaging, are limited by low resolution, interference by intervening structures, or long image acquisition times. Endoscopy provides good resolution of mucosal structures but gives little information about the underlying wall.

The combination of ultrasound and endoscopy provides a method for obtaining information about the gastrointestinal wall not provided by any other imaging technique. In this chapter, the principles of ultrasound interaction with tissue and specifically a layered structure such as the gastrointestinal wall will be outlined. The interpretation of ultrasound images of the normal esophagus, stomach, duodenum, and colon will be discussed. Finally, the various endoscopic ultrasound imaging systems that can be used to image the gastrointestinal wall will be reviewed.

PHYSICAL INTERACTION OF ULTRASOUND AND TISSUE

Ultrasound transducers emit a short-duration acoustic wave at a specified frequency(f) and wavelength. The wave propagates through a media at a velocity(c) that is characteristic of the media. The velocity of a medium is related to its stiffness (estimated by the bulk modulus K) and density (ρ) by the following equation:

$$c = (K/\rho)^{1/2}.$$

The acoustic velocity of most soft tissue depends on the magnitude of the bulk modulus, or stiffness, because the density is relatively constant. Stiffer tissues have a higher acoustic velocity. The characteristic acoustical impedance (Z) of a medium is related to its velocity and density by the relationship $Z = \rho c$.

Insight into how an echo is produced is gained by considering an acoustical wave propagating through a multilayered medium. The simplest case is a structure with two homogeneous layers that have characteristic acoustical impedances Z_1 and Z_2. Acoustic energy is reflected whenever a propagating wave encounters a change in acoustic impedance. Therefore, a reflected wave, or echo, will occur at the boundary between layers. The magnitude of the created echo is given by the reflection coefficient (R), which is simply the ratio of magni-

Table 3-1. Estimated acoustical properties of some biological media[33].

Media	Velocity	Density	Impedance	Attenuation coefficient
	C $(10^3\ \mathrm{m/s})$	ρ $(10^3\ \mathrm{kg/m^3})$	Z $(10^6\ \mathrm{kg/m^2 s})$	α at 1 MHz (Np/cm)
Blood	1.56	1.06	1.62	.02[12]
Fat	1.46–1.47	.92	1.35	.07[12]
Kidney	1.56	1.04	1.62	.033[14]
Liver	1.54–1.58	1.06	1.64–1.68	.1–.15[9]
Muscle	1.55–1.63	1.07	1.65–1.74	.18–.25[9]
Rectal wall	–	–	–	.07[12]
0.9% Saline				
at 20°	1.499	1.01	1.51	–
at 37°	1.560	1.01	1.58	–
Water				
at 20°	1.482	1.00	1.48	.00022[23]
at 37°	1.523	1.00	1.523	–

tudes of the incident and reflected waves. This reflection coefficient is related to the acoustical impedance of the media on both sides of the boundary by the following equation:

$$R = (Z_2 - Z_1)/(Z_2 + Z_1)$$

Layers with the largest differences in acoustical impedance have the largest reflection coefficient and therefore the largest amplitude of the reflected echo. The velocity of propagation, density, acoustic impedance, and attenuation for several types of biological media are listed in Table 3-1 (10, 12, 14, 23, 33).

The intestinal wall comprises four layers: mucosa, submucosa, muscularis propria, and serosa. If these layers were of different acoustical impedance but completely homogeneous within each layer, we would expect to see echoes only at the boundaries between layers. This is not the case for at least two reasons. First, roughness or waviness of the boundary region increases the duration or thickness of the boundary echo. Second, nonhomogeneity within a tissue layer will cause the acoustic wave to scatter energy, producing continuous echoes throughout the tissue layer. Areas with the largest nonhomogeneity in acoustical impedance will be the most echogenic.

Collagen and fat in the submucosa and subserosal regions of the gastrointestinal tract may be responsible for the echogenicity of these layers. Collagen fibers are stiff and have a high bulk modulus (9). The amplitude of scattered acoustic energy has been correlated with the collagen concentration of brain, heart, kidney, and tendon (19). The gastrointestinal submucosa contains abundant collagen and occasionally some fat. The subserosal area of the bowel often contains fat. Fat within tissue is also known to produce high amplitude echoes (29). Thus, collagen and fat could account for the echogenic nature of the submucosa and subserosal region of the bowel.

Attenuation of acoustical energy within the intestinal wall also may contribute to the form of the ultrasound image because echoes arising from tissue further from the transducer will be attenuated more. Attenuation is caused by energy loss owing to scattering and tissue absorption. The degree of attenuation is related both to the attenuation coefficient (α) and to the thickness of a tissue by the following equation:

$$I_x = I_o\, e^{-2\alpha x}$$

where I_o is the intensity of the incident wave, and I_x is the intensity of the wave after it travels a distance x through a medium with an attenuation coefficient α.

The attenuation coefficient of a tissue varies with temperature, pH, ultrasonic frequency, and tissue constituents (34). Most attenuation within a tissue occurs at or below the macromolecular level (8). The collagen content of a tissue also correlates with the level of attenuation (18). Attenuation within the submucosa of the intestine may produce difficulty in imaging deeper layers of the wall. In addition, the increased attenuation and reduced penetration seen with higher frequencies may limit attempts to increase resolution by using very high imaging frequencies.

INTERPRETATION OF GASTROINTESTINAL WALL IMAGES

Several layers are seen on both histological sections and ultrasound images of the gastrointestinal wall. The simplest interpretation of the layers visible in ultrasound images is that they correspond directly to the histological layers. This interpretation led several early investigators to conclude that the first echogenic layer corresponded to mucosa, the second echolucent layer represented muscularis mucosae, the third or central echogenic layer corresponded to submucosa, the fourth echolucent layer was muscularis propria, and the fifth echogenic layer was produced by serosa and subserosal fat (5, 30).

This interpretation of the ultrasound image was oversimplified. The second echolucent layer was too thick to represent the very thin muscularis mucosae (1). These interpretations often were based on comparisons made between in vivo images and in vitro histological sections (5). At best, the images were made of a resected specimen and compared with the histological section of the approximate area of tissue that was imaged (30). Even when in vitro images were compared with the histology of what was thought to be the same tissue, interpretation was still difficult. The second layer continued to be interpreted by some investigators as the muscularis mucosae (30, 31).

As discussed earlier, echoes are generated when the ultrasound beam encounters a change in the acoustical impedance of the tissue through which it is passing. One might expect the boundary between two layers of the gastrointestinal wall to produce such an echo. This reasoning led to the hypothesis that the appearance of echogenic layers on images of the gut wall (layers 1, 3, 5, see below) were produced by these boundaries (2, 4). This explanation did not account for any echoes produced by scattering within the tissue itself, however.

We hypothesized that better interpretation of ultrasound images could be made if ultrasound images of the gastrointestinal wall could be compared precisely with the corresponding histological section of the imaged tissue (25). Many factors must be controlled to accomplish such a comparison. Excised tissue must be prepared, mounted, and scanned in a manner that preserves as much as possible the in vivo ultrasonic characteristics of a tissue. The position of the transducer and scan plane in space must be known precisely to assure that the tissue imaged is the same as that that will be later sectioned for histology. Finally, a well-controlled method of obtaining the histological section from the tissue is required so that the sectioned region corresponds exactly to the imaged region.

We developed a system to obtain ultrasound images and histological sections in this way and have used this system to image resected gastrointestinal wall specimens (15, 16). These in vitro studies have aided the interpretation of normal wall structure, which appears below. This interpretation applies to ultrasound images made with 7.5 to 10-MHz transducers. Lower frequency transducers may not provide as much detail and higher frequency transducers may give greater structural resolution. Most investigators in this field now agree on the interpretation outlined below (1, 3, 15, 16, 17, 20, 22, 26–28, 32).

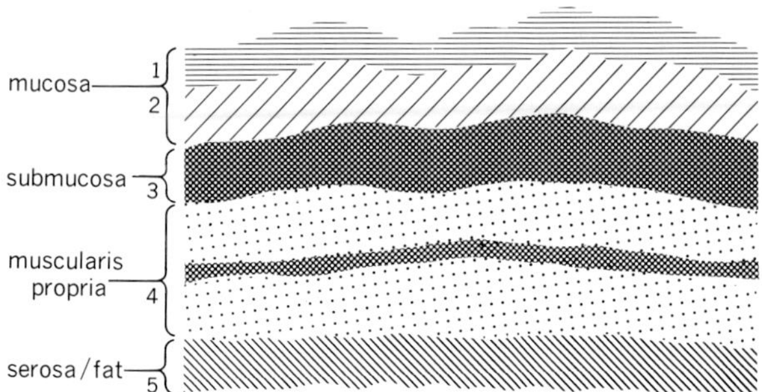

Fig. 3-1. The layered appearance of ultrasound images of the gastrointestinal wall and how these layers correspond to the histology of the wall. The layers are numbered according to the description in the text.

BASIC GASTROINTESTINAL WALL STRUCTURE

Five major layers are seen on most images throughout the GI tract. Although there may be small regional differences, the interpretation of the five layers is the same from the esophagus through the rectum. A diagram of the layers seen on ultrasound images, the numbering of these layers, and how they correspond to histology is shown in Fig. 3-1. Regional differences are outlined by organ in the following sections.

The first echogenic layer corresponds with the interface between the transducer or fluid surrounding the transducer and the mucosa. The second echolucent area corresponds with the deep mucosa and possibly the muscularis mucosae. The third and most echogenic layer is produced by the submucosa. The fourth layer is echolucent and corresponds with the muscularis propria. The fifth layer is echogenic and corresponds with the serosa and subserosal fat, and possibly the interface with the surrounding tissue.

Esophagus

The esophageal wall is thin and may be difficult to examine with existing ultrasound endoscopes because of compression by the balloon surrounding the transducer (3, 6, 22). The primary five layers usually can be seen but may appear thin. Caution must be exercised in interpreting layer thickness if a balloon is used because of the effects of tissue compression. The esophagus does not have a serosal covering; however, the adventitia and surrounding fat comprise the outer echogenic layer.

Stomach

An example of the sonogram and corresponding histological section of a segment of gastric wall and pylorus is shown in Fig. 3-2. The second layer often is thicker in the stomach, particularly if there is incomplete distension during examination (3). Occasionally a very thin line is seen within the second layer near the third layer. This line may be produced by the muscularis mucosae or perhaps owing to the interface between the lamina propria and muscularis mucosae (1, 15). Careful correlation of ultrasound with histology and perhaps higher frequency transducers are needed to define this area better.

The fourth layer of the stomach wall may contain a few echoes although it remains generally echo poor. These few echoes may be created by the oblique muscle layer within the gastric muscularis propria. The fundus and body of the stomach may be slightly thinner than the antrum. Thickening of the muscularis propria layer in the region of the pylorus also may be noted (Fig. 3-2).

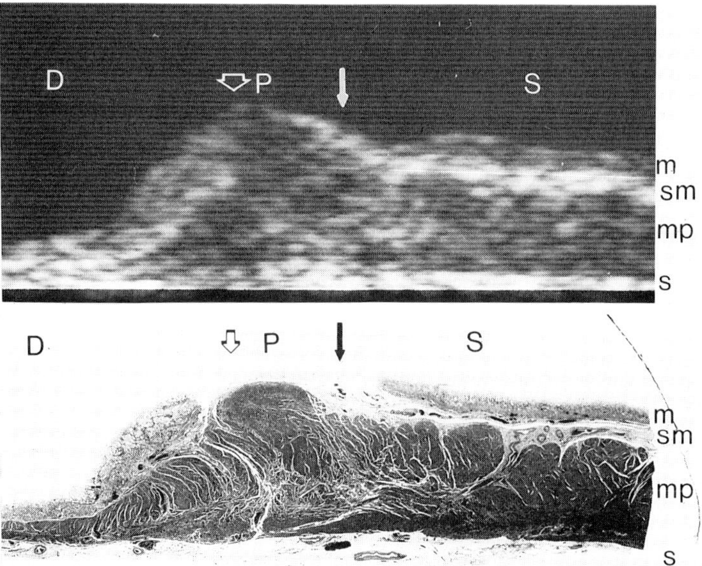

Fig. 3-2. The ultrasound image (*top*) of normal gastroduodenal wall is compared with the histological section (*bottom*) of the same area of tissue. Mucosa (m), submucosa (sm), muscularis propria (mp), and serosa (s) are clearly shown. Layers 1 and 2 on the image are absent where the mucosa has been removed (arrows). Layers 1, 2, and 3 are absent on the image where both mucosa and submucosa have been removed (open arrows). Duodenum (D), pylorus (P), and stomach (S) are all seen in this example.

Duodenum

The duodenal layers often are thin and difficult to visualize because of the effect of compression by the transducer. This compression, along with difficulty orienting the transducer perpendicular to the wall, may cause only three layers to be seen (3). However, careful orientation and limited balloon distension allows the basic five layers to be visualized (32).

Colon

Five layers usually are seen well in the colon. An echogenic line often is seen within the fourth layer when the US beam is parallel to the taenia coli. This line corresponds with an area of connective tissue between the inner and outer layers of the muscularis propria (1, 3). The thickness of the outer layer varies depending on how much subserosal fat is present.

Rectum

The rectum is similar in ultrasonographic appearance to the colon (1, 3, 22). The fourth layer may be slightly thicker, corresponding with the thicker rectal muscularis propria. There are no taenia coli in the rectum, so the inner and outer portions of the muscularis propria can be seen in all areas. The area between these two muscle layers usually is visible as an echogenic line within layer 4. In the most distal rectum, layer 4 is thicker where the inner circular fibers form the internal anal sphincter (3). An example of an ultrasound image of rectal wall and the corresponding histological section illustrates the relationship of the rectal wall layers to each other (Fig. 3-3).

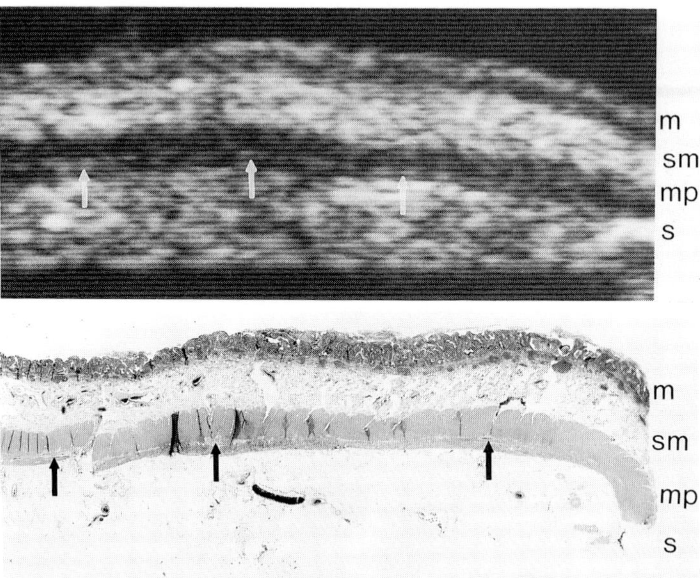

Fig. 3-3. The ultrasound image (*top*) and corresponding histological section of a segment of rectum from a patient with ulcerative colitis is shown. Mucosa (m), submucosa (sm), muscularis propria (mp), connective tissue between the two layers of muscularis propria (arrows), and serosa/subserosa (s) are shown.

METHODS OF GASTROINTESTINAL WALL ULTRASOUND

Several systems that combine endoscopy and ultrasound have been used to image the intestinal wall (24). Linear arrays and mechanical sector scanners have been attached to endoscopes for this purpose. Linear array-endoscope combinations have 32 to 64 individual elements that are used to image a field approximately 3 cm wide and 6 cm deep (7, 11, 26). The rectilinear format limits the width of the distal field but provides a well-oriented and wide proximal field, two important factors when examining the intestinal wall. Multiple coaxial cables are necessary to activate the multiple array elements, limiting miniaturization of the endoscope. A 4 cm long array has been positioned at the tip of the endoscope (7) or on the shaft of the endoscope several centimeters proximal to the tip (11). Entry into the descending duodenum is easier with the second design.

Mechanical sector scanners also have been incorporated by several groups into endoscopes (30, 35). These devices do not require multiple coaxial cables. Ultrasonic frequencies of 5, 7.5, and 10 MHz have been used. The transducer rotates in the tip of the endoscope, producing a sector scan with either a 180° or 360° field of view. Using fluid as an interface or standoff, this system can provide excellent images of the intestinal wall and surrounding structures (32).

Although electrically simpler than an array system, the mechanical sector scanning systems have some limitations. The transducer is rotated by turning a cable inside the endoscope, adding to the complexity and size of the instrument. The motor used to rotate the transducer adds weight to the endoscope. The endoscope must be either side- or oblique-viewing because the optics must end before its tip to provide space for the transducer. As with the other systems, the tip of the endoscope is rigid for a length of up to 4 cm. This may cause difficulty in passing the instrument into the descending duodenum.

Devices using both linear arrays and mechanical sector scanners have been used for transrectal imaging (21, 22). Most of these devices are passed blindly into the rectum because they do not have an optical system. These systems have been used primarily in the rectum to stage rectal cancer, and to image the prostate, bladder, and uterus. Passing an ultrasound transducer more proximally into the colon thus far has been impossible.

Several problems with currently available ultrasound endoscopes may be clarified with further study. Identifying and characterizing these problems may lead to a new system design for imaging the intestinal wall. Current devices are expensive, limiting availability and the ability of a center to have several echoendoscopes on hand. If either the ultrasound system or the optical system breaks, an instrument may be unavailable while repairs are made. Interpretation of images also can be difficult. One must learn ultrasound interpretation of images obtained at unpredictable angles. Finally, with the side- or oblique-viewing systems it is not possible to pass the device into the colon where end-viewing is a necessary prerequisite. We have recently described an ultrasound probe for imaging the gastrointestinal wall (25A). This probe passes down the biopsy channel of conventional upper endoscopes and colonoscopes, obviating some of the problems outlined above.

SUMMARY

Endoscopic ultrasonography offers new diagnostic information about the gastrointestinal tract wall. Understanding the physics of ultrasound and its interaction with a layered structure aids in the interpretation of images. Images of the gastrointestinal tract wall are similar throughout its course although there are small regional differences. Further careful correlation of ultrasound images with tissue structure may provide additional information about the ultrasound image. Modifications in existing instruments or new methods of applying ultrasound to the gastrointestinal wall also may increase the diagnostic utility of endoscopic ultrasound.

Acknowledgement
This work was supported in part by a grant from the United States National Institutes of Health (RO1 AM34814) and by equipment from Advanced Technology Laboratories, Bellevue, Washington, USA.

References
1. Aibe T, Fuji T, Okita K, Takemoto T: A fundamental study of normal layer structure of the gastrointestinal wall visualized by endoscopic ultrasonography. Scand J Gastroenterol 21 (Suppl 123): 1-5, 1986.
2. Bolondi L, Casanova P, Bertarelli C, Santi V, Caletti G, Labo G: In vitro investigation of the sonographic appearance of normal gastric wall. Gastroenterology 86: 1031, 1984.
3. Bolondi L, Caletti G, Casanova P, Villanacci V, Grigioni W, Labo G: Problems and variations in the interpretation of the ultrasound feature of the normal upper and lower GI tract wall. Scand J Gastroenterol 21 (Suppl 123): 16-26, 1986.
4. Boscaini M, Montori A: Transrectal ultrasonography: Interpretation of normal intestinal wall structure for the preoperative staging of rectal cancer. Scan J Gastroenterol 21 (Suppl 123): 87-98, 1986.
5. Caletti G, Bolondi L, Labo G: Ultrasonic endoscopy—the gastrointestinal wall. Scand J Gastroenterol 19 (Suppl 102): 5-8, 1984.
6. Caletti G, Bolondi L, Zani L, Labo G: Technique of endoscopic ultrasonography investigation: Esophagus, stomach, and duodenum. Scand J Gastroenterol 21 (Suppl 123): 1-5, 1986.
7. DiMagno, EP, Regan PT, Clain JE, James EM, Buxton JL: Human endoscopic ultrasonography. Gastroenterology 83: 824-829, 1983.

8.   Edmonds PD: The molecular basis of ultrasonic absorption in proteins. In Takashima S, Postow E (eds): The Interaction of Acoustical and Electromagnetic Fields with Biological Systems. Alan R. Liss Inc., New York, 1982, pp 157–165.

9.   Fields S, Dunn F: Correlation of echographic visualizability of tissue with biological composition and physiological state. J Acoust Soc Am 54: 809–812, 1973.

10.   Goldman DE, Hueter TF: Tabular data of the velocity and absorption of high-frequency sound in mammalian tissue. J Acoust Soc Am 28: 35–37, 1956.

11.   Gordon SJ, Rifkin MD, Goldberg BB: Endosonographic evaluation of mural abnormalities of the upper gastrointestinal tract. Gastrointest Endosc 32: 193–198, 1986.

12.   Goss SA, Johnston RL, Dunn F: Comprehensive compilation of empirical ultrasonic properties of mammalian tissues. J Acoust Soc Am 64: 423–447, 1978.

13.   Goss SA, Frizzell LA, Dunn F, Dines KA: Dependence of the ultrasonic properties of biological tissue on constituent proteins. J Acoust Soc Am 67: 1041–1044, 1980.

14.   Goss SA, Johnston RL, Dunn F: Compilation of empirical ultrasonic properties of mammalian tissues II. J Acoust Soc Am 68: 93–108, 1980.

15.   Kimmey MB, Silverstein FE, Haggitt RC, Mack LA, Nyberg DA, Martin RC: Ultrasound (US) imaging of gastrointestinal wall: New insights from comparative histologic studies. Gastroenterology 90: 1493, 1986.

16.   Kimmey MB, Silverstein FE, Haggitt RC, Shuman WP, Mack LA, Rohrmann CA, Moss AA, Franklin DW: Cross sectional imaging method: A system to compare ultrasound, computed tomography, and magnetic resonance with histologic findings. Invest Radiol 22: 227–231, 1987.

17.   Machi J, Takeda J, Sigel B, Kakegawa T: Normal stomach wall and gastric cancer: Evaluation with high-resolution operative US. Radiology 159: 85–87, 1986.

18.   Pohlhammer JD, O'Brien WD: The relationship between ultrasonic attenuation and speed in tissue and the constituents: Water, collagen, protein, and fat. In Fullerton GD, Zagzebski JA (eds): Medical Physics of CT and Ultrasound: Tissue Imaging and Characterization. American Institute of Physics, New York, 1980, pp 408–435.

19.   Pohlhammer J, O'Brien WD Jr: Dependence of the ultrasonic scatter coefficient on collagen concentration in mammalian tissues. J Acoust Soc Am 69: 282–285, 1981.

20.   Rifkin MD, Gordon SJ, Goldberg BB: Sonographic examination of the mediastinum and upper abdomen by fiberoptic gastroscope. Radiology 151: 175–180, 1984.

21.   Rifkin MD, McGlynn ET, Marks G: Endorectal sonographic prospective staging of rectal cancer. Scand J Gastroenterol 21: 99–103, 1986.

22.   Saitog N, Okui K, Sarashina H, Suzuki M, Arai T, Nunomura M: Evaluation of echographic diagnosis of rectal cancer using intrarectal ultrasonic examination. Dis Col Rectum 29: 234–242, 1986.

23.   Selfridge AR: Approximate material properties in isotropic materials. IEEE Trans Sonics Ultrasonics 32: 381–394, 1985.

24.   Silverstein F, Giuliani D, Daigle R: Endoscopic ultrasound. Acta Endoscopica 13: 1–9, 1983.

25.   Silverstein F, Kimmey M, Martin R, Haggitt R, Mack L, Moss A, Franklin D: Ultrasound and the intestinal wall: Experimental methods. Scand J Gastroenterol 21 (Suppl 123): 34–40, 1986.

25A.   Silverstein FE, Martin RW, Kimmey MB: The endoscopic echo probe: A new approach to imaging the intestinal wall. Gastrointest Endosc 33: 178, 1987.

26.   Strohm WD, Classen M: Benign lesions of the upper GI tract by means of endoscopic ultrasonography. Scand J Gastroenterol 21 (Suppl 123): 41–46, 1986.

27.   Takemoto T, Aibe T, Fuji T, Okita K: Endoscopic ultrasonography. Clin Gastroenterol 15: 305–319, 1986.

28.   Tanaka Y, Yasuda K, Aibe T, Fuji T, Kawai K: Anatomical and pathological aspects in ultrasonic endoscopy for GI tract. Scand J Gastroenterol 19 (Suppl 94): 43–50, 1984.

29.   Taylor KJW, Jacobson P, Talmont CA, Winters R: Manual of Ultrasonography. Churchill Livingstone, New York, 1980, p 11.

30.   Tio TL, Tytgat GNJ: Endoscopic ultrasonography in the assessment of intra- and transmural infiltration of tumours in the oesophagus, stomach, and papilla of Vater and in the detection of extraesophageal lesions. Endoscopy 16: 203–210, 1984.

31.   Tio TL, Tytgat GNJ: Endoscopic ultrasonography of normal and pathologic upper gastrointestinal wall structure. Comparison of studies in vivo and in vitro with histology. Scan J Gastroenterol 21 (Suppl 123): 27–33, 1986.

32.   Tio TL, Tytgat GNJ: Atlas of Transintestinal Ultrasound. Mur-Kostverloren, Aalsmere, The Netherlands, 1986.

33.   Wells, PNT: Basic physics. In deVlieger M, Holmes JH, Kratochwil A, Kazner E, Kraus R,

Kossoff G., Poujol J, Strandness DE (eds): Handbook of Clinical Ultrasound. John Wiley & Sons, New York, 1978, pp 15–23.
34. Wells PNT: Propagation of ultrasonic waves through tissue. In Fullerton GD, Zagzebski JA (eds): Medical Physics of CT and Ultrasound: Tissue Imaging and Characterization. American Institute of Physics, New York, 1980, pp 367–387.
35. Yasuda K, Nakajima M, Kawai K: Endoscopic ultrasonography in the diagnosis of submucosal tumor of the upper digestive tract. Scand J Gastroenterol 21 (Suppl 123): 59–67, 1986.

4

Benign Lesions of the Gastrointestinal Tract

Tsuyoshi Aibe and Tadayoshi Takemoto

Endoscopic ultrasonography (EUS) is the latest diagnostic procedure in the field of gastroenterology and gives us much information regarding the gastrointestinal tract and pancreatobiliary tree (2). Since 1980, we have investigated the diagnostic usefulness of EUS in 615 cases: 290 cases of gastrointestinal disease, 257 cases of pancreatobiliary disorders, and 68 other disorders. In this chapter, we will clarify the value of this technique for the diagnosis of benign lesions of the gastrointestinal tract.

SUBJECTS AND METHODS

Table 4-1 shows the gastrointestinal disease cases in which we performed EUS. Benign diseases of the gastrointestinal tract were investigated in 107 cases, including 33 cases of submucosal tumor and 25 cases of peptic ulcer. In this series we used two ultrasonic endoscopes. One was a radial scanning instrument developed in cooperation with Olympus Optical Co. and Aloka Co. (Tokyo); the other was a linear-array device made by Toshiba Medical Co. in cooperation with Machida Co. (Tokyo) (2).

Premedication for EUS is the same as that for gastrointestinal endoscopy. In the investigation of lesions by EUS, either the liquid-filled method or the balloon method was adopted (2).

Table 4-1. Cases of gastrointestinal diseases in which EUS was performed.

	Benign lesion	Malignant lesion
Esophagus	21	33
Stomach	62	125
Duodenum	8	9
Colon	16	16
Total	107	183

LAYER STRUCTURE OF THE GASTROINTESTINAL WALL VISUALIZED BY EUS

The echo levels in the gastrointestinal wall usually can be divided by EUS into five layers (1). A diagram of the histological structure of the gastrointestinal wall as visualized by EUS is shown in Fig. 4-1. With five layers of the gastrointestinal wall, the first hyperechoic and hypoechoic layer correspond to the mucosa, the next hyperechoic layer (the third layer) is the submucosa, and the fourth, the hypoechoic layer, corresponds to the muscularis propria. The first hyperechoic layer is a border echo demonstrated inside the mucosa. The fifth, the hyperechoic layer, comprises the serosa (or the adventitia) and a border echo visualized outside the serosa (or the adventitia). The five-layer structure of the gastric wall visualized by the most modern ultrasonic endoscope (GF-UM 2/EU-M 2; Olympus Optical Co. and Aloka Co.) is shown on the left echogram of Fig. 4-1.

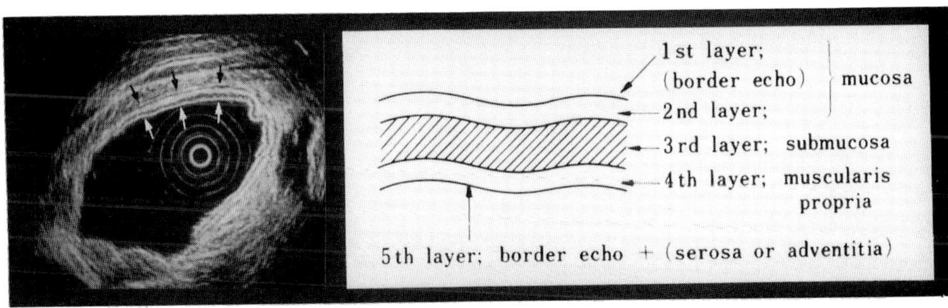

Fig. 4-1. Diagram of the histological structure of the five layers of the gastrointestinal wall as visualized by EUS is shown. On the left, the five-layer structure of the gastric wall (arrows) demonstrated by the radial scanning ultrasonic endoscope with a 10 MHz transducer is shown.

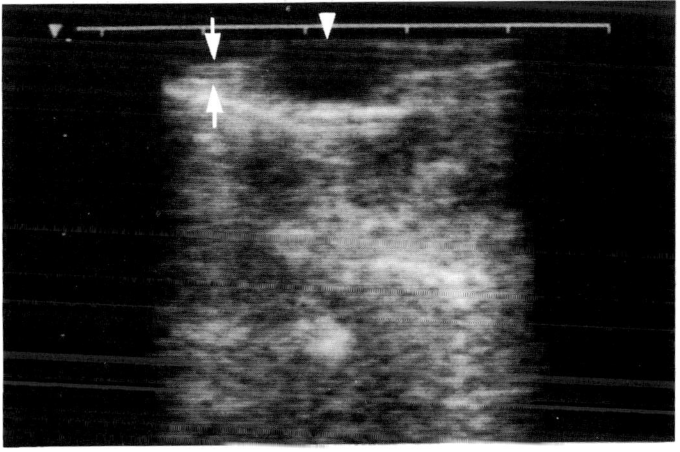

Fig. 4-2. The arrowhead indicates a submucosal tumor of the esophagus visualized by the linear-arrayed ultrasonic endoscope with a 5-MHz transducer. Five-layer structure of the esophageal wall is seen between the two opposing arrows.

SUBMUCOSAL TUMOR

Twenty-six submucosal tumor cases were in the stomach, five were in the esophagus, and two were in the sigmoid colon. Figs. 4-2 through 4-7 are examples of endoscopic ultrasonic findings in the gastrointestinal submucosal tumor and the external compression to the gastrointestinal tract by other organs.

Normally it is easy to distinguish a submucosal tumor from extracompression on the tract by EUS. Moreover, the genetic tissue of the submucosal tumor in the gastrointestinal wall

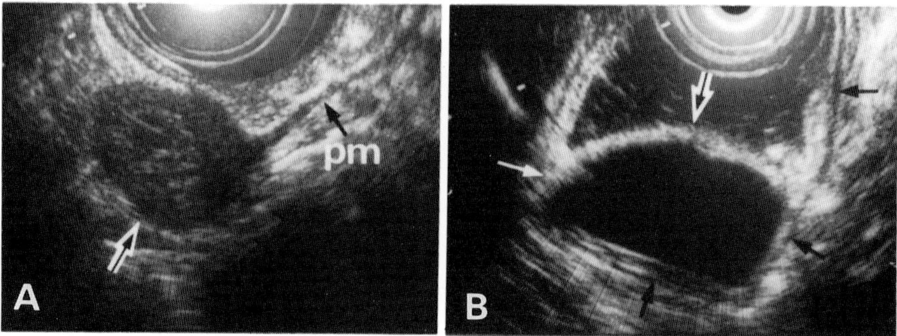

Fig. 4-3. Two cases of the gastric submucosal tumor demonstrated by the radial scanning instrument with a 10-MHz probe. **A.** Black-white arrow points toward a solid tumor that grew from the muscularis propria (pm) toward the outside. **B.** Black-white arrow indicates a submucosal cyst that existed in the submucosal tissue and grew toward the inside. Black arrows show the fourth layer of the gastric wall (muscularis propria) without change, the white arrow indicates the third layer (submucosa).

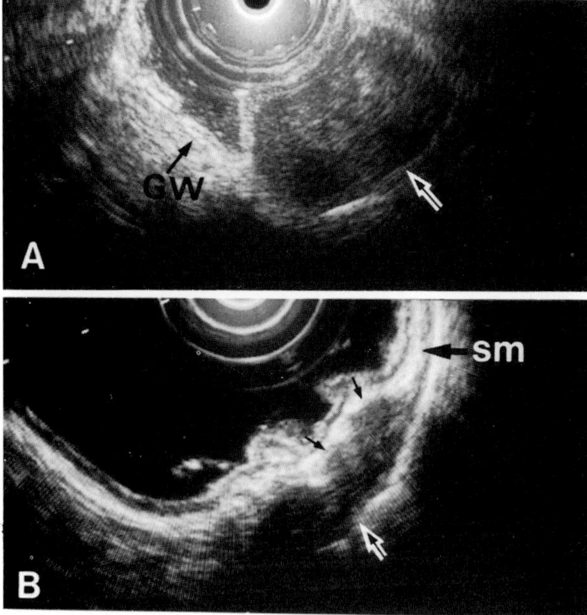

Fig. 4-4. Histological presentation of gastric leiomyoma (A) and gastric leiomyosarcoma (B). Black-white arrows in A and B indicate the lesion. It is difficult to distinguish a leiomyoma from a leiomyosarcoma with the internal-echo pattern of the tumor. However, changes of the layer structure as shown in B (black arrows) demonstrate the malignant invasion. GW, gastric wall; sm, submucosa.

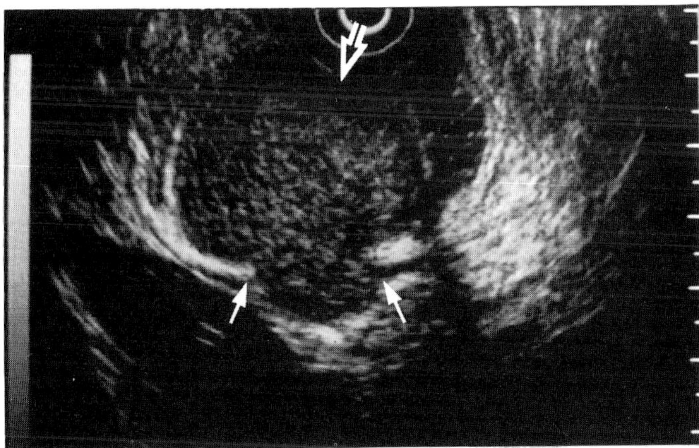

Fig. 4-5. Histological presentation of a gastric leiomyoblastoma (black-white arrow). The destruction of the layer structure of the gastric wall (white arrows) indicates a malignant submucosal tumor.

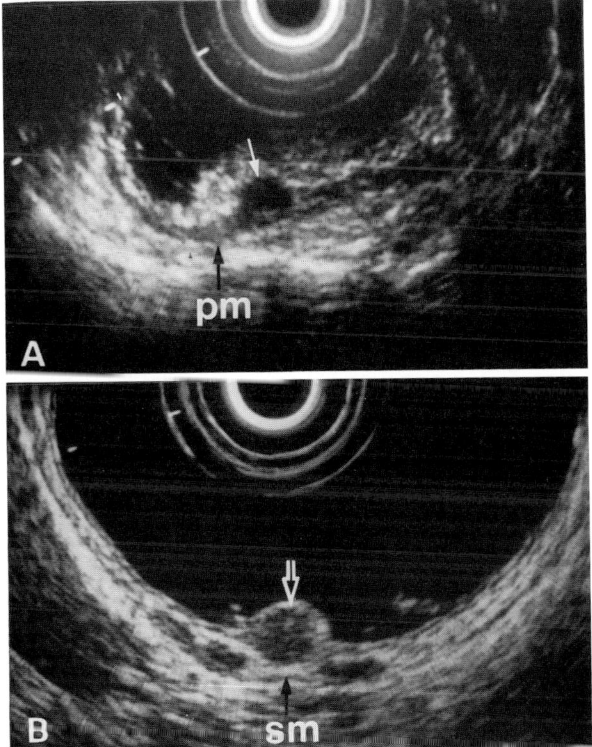

Fig. 4-6. Endoscopic ultrasonic findings of cases diagnosed as submucosal tumors of the sigmoid colon by usual endoscopic observation. **A.** White arrow points toward a tumor emanating from the muscularis propria (pm). **B.** Black-white arrow indicates a tumor existing in the mucosa and the submucosa (sm) that is compressed toward the muscularis propria by the tumor. Using EUS, **A** was diagnosed as a submucosal tumor, whereas **B** was diagnosed as an intramucosal tumor. **B** proved to be carcinoid by histological findings after biopsy.

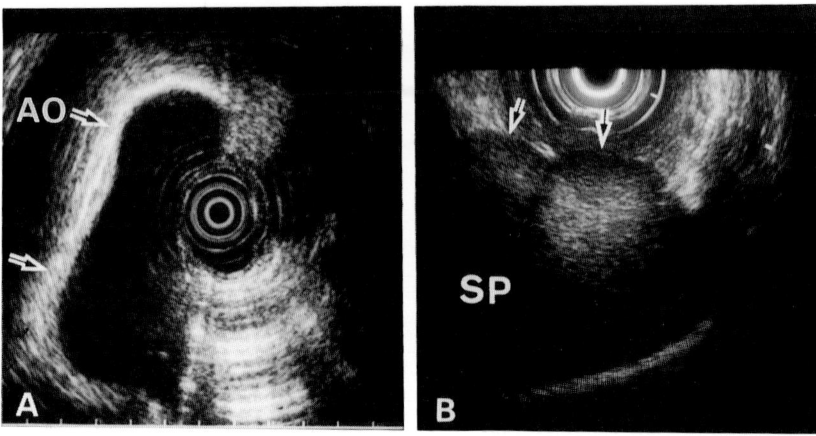

Fig. 4-7. Endoscopic ultrasonograms of two cases of the external compression to the upper GI tract by other organs. **A.** Extracompression to the esophagus by the descending aorta (AO). **B.** Extracompression to the gastric fornix (arrows) by the spleen (SP).

Table 4-2. A comparison with EUS findings and histological findings of the depth of the resected gastric ulcer specimen.

Case No.	EUS	Histology
1	Submucosa	Submucosa
2	ss-s	ss-s
3	ss-s	ss-s
4	ss-s	ss-s
5	ss-s	ss-s
6	ss-s	ss-s
7	Penetration	Penetration

ss-s: Subserosa-serosa.

Table 4-3. Cases of gastric ulcer in which EUS was performed.

Case No.	Age	Sex	Depth (EUS)	Therapy		Healing period (wks)
1	72	M	Submucosa	Ranitidine		6
2	59	M	Submucosa	Cimetidine		8
3	29	F	Muscle	Famotidine		4
4	69	F	Muscle	Omeprazole		4
5	58	F	Muscle	Ranitidine		5
6	60	F	Muscle	Ranitidine		6
7	40	F	ss-s	AG-1749		6
8	51	M	ss-s	Cimetidine		4
9	70	M	ss-s	Omeprazole		8
10	47	F	ss-s	Famotidine		10
11	32	M	ss-s	Cimetidine		10
12	72	F	ss-s	Ranitidine		12
13	39	M	ss-s	Cimetidine	⟶	operation
14	40	M	ss-s	Cimetidine	⟶	operation
15	48	M	ss-s	Ranitidine	⟶	operation
16	52	M	ss-s	Cimetidine	⟶	operation
17	74	F	ss-s	Ranitidine	⟶	operation
18	53	M	Penetration	Ranitidine	⟶	operation
19	68	M	Penetration	Ranitidine	⟶	16 weeks
20	63	M	Penetration	Ranitidine	⟶	18 weeks

ss-s: Subserosa-serosa.

can be decided by studying the relationship between the tumor and the layer structure, and the growth direction of the tumor is determined by the same method. Regarding the differential diagnosis of malignant and benign submucosal tumors, it is thought that the only important finding is if the layer structure of the gastrointestinal wall has been destroyed by the tumor.

PEPTIC ULCER

Gastric Ulcer

EUS has provided much information regarding the peptic ulcer. An accurate diagnosis of the ulcer depth and a prediction of the healing process can now be made by this method.

Table 4-2 compares EUS findings with the histological findings by using resected gastric ulcer specimens. The EUS findings give an accurate diagnosis of the depth of the gastric ulcer in all cases. The relationship between the depth of the gastric ulcer diagnosed by EUS and the

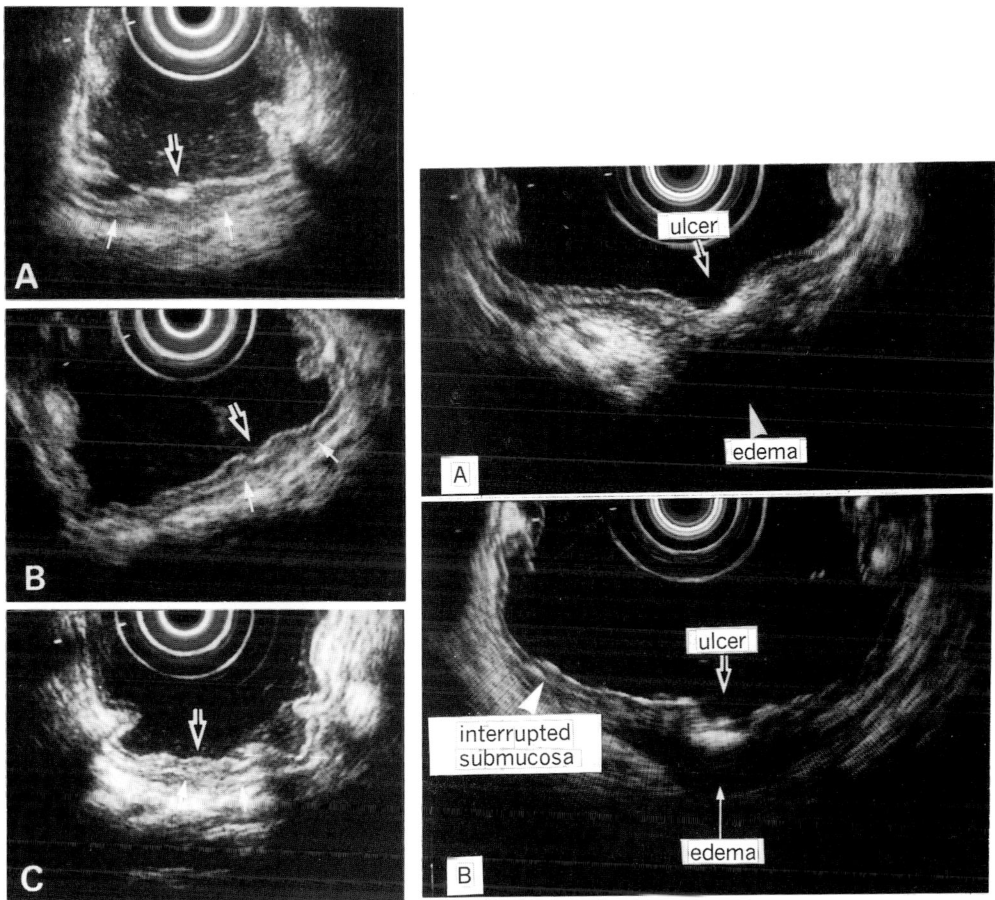

Fig. 4-8.   Fig. 4-9.

Fig. 4-8. Endoscopic ultrasonic findings of the healing process of a gastric ulcer (black-white arrows), of which the ulcer depth was diagnosed by EUS to be in the muscularis propria. White arrows in **A, B,** and **C** indicate the interrupted submucosa. **A.** Active stage. **B.** healing stage **C.** scar stage.

Fig. 4-9. Endoscopic ultrasonic findings of typical cases of H_2-blocker resistant gastric ulcers. Edematous swelling remains at the bottom of the gastric wall, although endoscopic observation revealed the ulcers to be in the healing stage (**A, B**). In **B**, the submucosa is interrupted far from the ulcer.

Table 4-4. Cases of duodenal ulcer in which EUS was performed.

Case No.	Age	Sex	Depth (EUS)	Therapy	Healing period (wks)
1	62	M	Submucosa	Ranitidine	2
2	74	M	Muscle	Omeprazole	4
3	20	M	ss-s	Emprostil	6
4	36	F	Penetration	Ranitidine	8
5	79	F	Penetration	Ranitidine	8

ss-s: Subserosa-serosa.

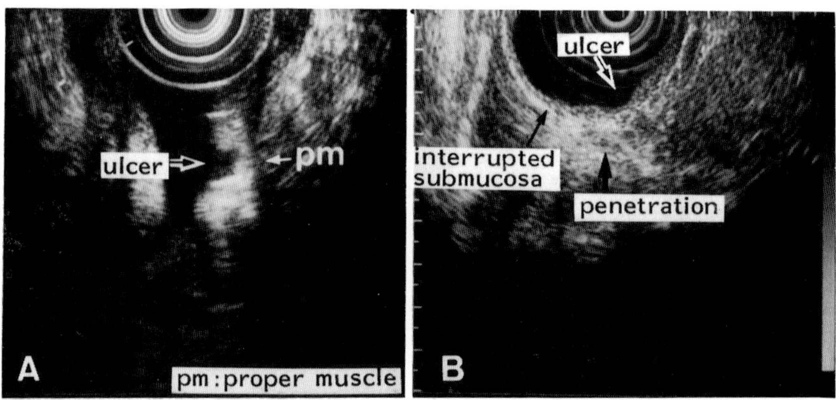

Fig. 4-10. Endoscopic ultrasonic findings of two cases with duodenal ulcer. **A** is an open ulcer, with its depth diagnosed in the muscularis propria (pm), because the muscularis propria was narrowed at the bottom of the ulcer. **B** is an ulcer scar; the interruption of the submucosa and the penetration to the extraduodenal wall are shown.

healing period is shown in Table 4-3. Fourteen cases were cured by conservative therapy, and six (case 13 to case 18) operated on surgically because of intractability or repeated recurrence.

Five of 14 cases treated with conservative therapy (cases 10 to 12 and 19 and 20) required treatment with H_2-blocker for more than eight weeks. If the "H_2-blocker resistant ulcer" is defined as an endoscopically proven ulcer that does not heal with least eight weeks treatment with the standard dose of H_2-blocker, characteristic findings of EUS in the cases of H_2-blocker resistant ulcer were as follows: The depth of these ulcers was beyond the muscularis propria and reached to the subserosa or serosa, or penetrated the gastric wall; edematous swelling remained in the bottom of the gastric wall even with the ulcer in the endoscopic healing stage; and the submucosa and the muscularis propria were interrupted at a point far from the ulcer in all five cases. This finding meant that an old healed ulcer with the depth beyond the muscularis propria coexisted around the current ulcer. Typical cases of gastric ulcer are shown in Figs. 4-8 and 4-9.

Duodenal Ulcer

EUS was performed in five cases of duodenal ulcer as shown in Table 4-4. All cases healed within eight weeks with medication. There was a tendency toward slow healing in deeper ulcers. Two typical cases with duodenal ulcer are shown in Fig. 4-10.

OTHERS

There were nine cases of esophageal varices and 17 cases of inflammatory disorders, including acute gastric mucosal lesion (AGML), giant rugae of the stomach, and ulcerative colitis.   A

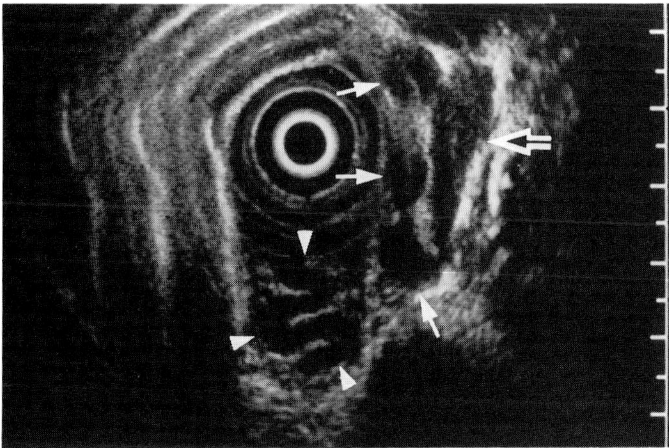

Fig. 4-11.   Endoscopic ultrasonic findings of esophageal varices.   Arrowheads point toward the winding and meandering varices in the esophageal wall.   White arrows indicate other varices in the esophageal wall, which connect to paraesophageal varices (black-white arrow).

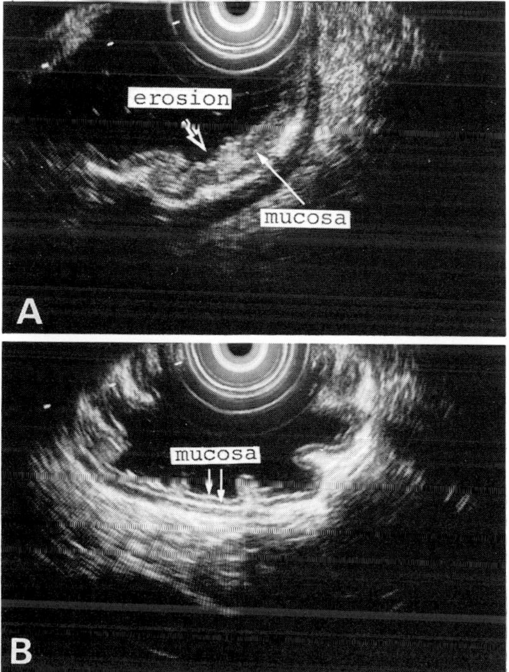

Fig. 4-12.   Acute gastric mucosal lesion (AGML).   **A.** The second layer of the gastric wall, which is a part of the mucosa, is thickened around an erosion.   **B.** Layer structure is intact at another part of the gastric wall without AGML in the same case as **A.**

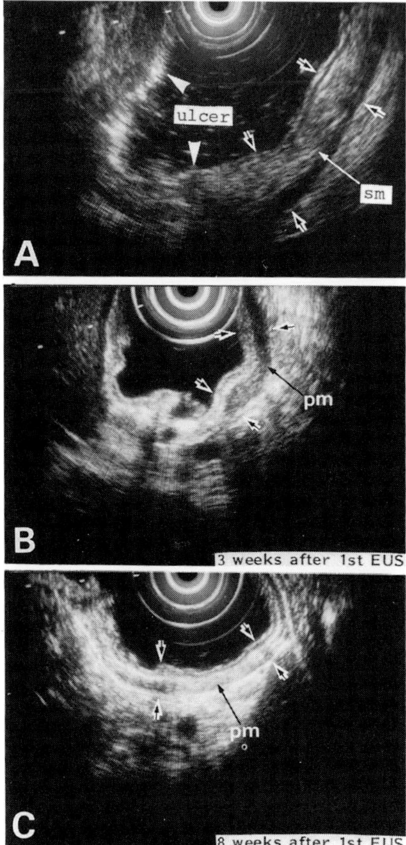

Fig. 4-13. Endoscopic ultrasonic findings of the healing process of AGML. **A.** Active stage. The entire gastric wall surrounding this ulcer was remarkably thickened; this wall (arrows) comprised mainly the third (submucosa, sm) and fourth layers (muscularis propria, pm). **B.** The stage at which inflammatory changes disappeared in the usual endoscopic observation. The deep tissue of the gastric wall (muscularis propria, pm) remained thickened. **C.** Healed stage. Gastric wall (arrows) recovered the normal layer structure by eight weeks after the first EUS.

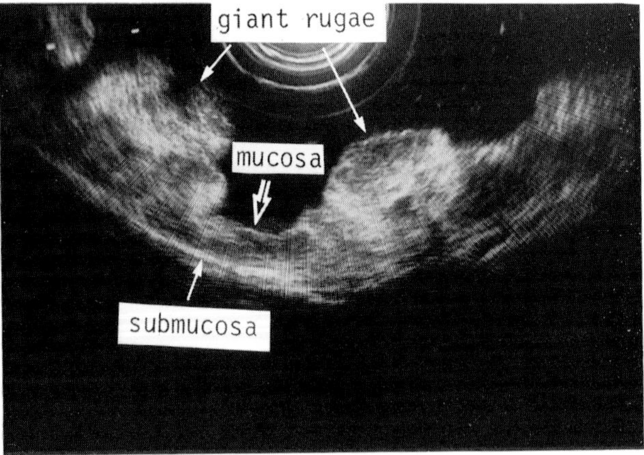

Fig. 4-14. Endoscopic ultrasonic findings of a case of Menétrier's disease. Giant folds comprised the remarkable swelling of the mucosa. The mucosa of the gastric wall, besides the folds, is also thickened.

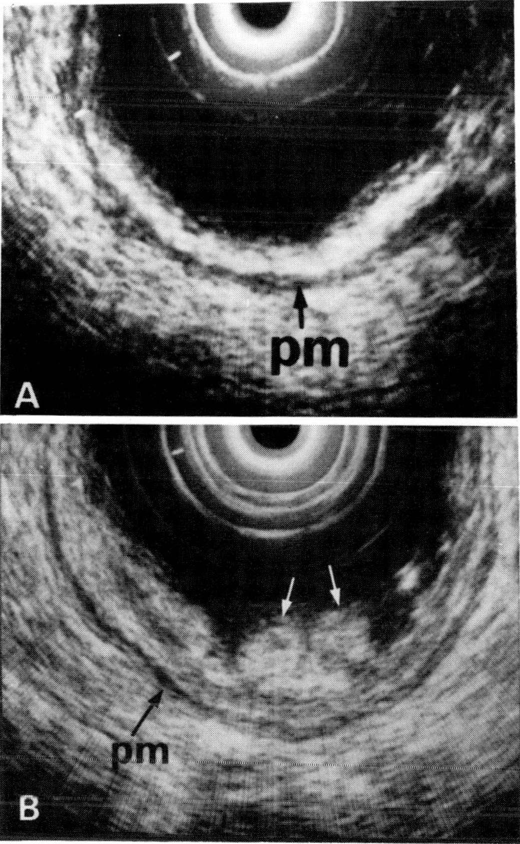

Fig. 4-15. Ulcerative colitis. It is a characteristic finding on echograms that the second and third layers are thickened. White arrows in **B** show the pseudopolyps. pm, muscularis propria.

typical case of esophageal varices is shown in Fig. 4-11. It has been reported that the accurate judgment of the effect of injection sclerotherapy to esophageal varices can be made by performing EUS before and after its therapy (3). Figs. 4-12 through 4-14 are endoscopic ultrasonic findings of AGML and giant rugae of the stomach.

In five cases of AGML, the differentiation between erosion and ulceration was clarified by EUS. With erosions, the second layer of the gastric wall, which is a part of the mucosa, was thickened around the erosions, whereas, in cases combined with ulcerations, the entire gastric wall surrounding the ulcerations was remarkably thickened; this thickened wall comprised mainly the swelling of the submucosa (third layer) and muscularis propria (fourth layer). Furthermore, EUS showed that the deep tissue of the gastric wall (muscularis propria) remained thickened even after the inflammatory changes disappeared in the usual endoscopic observation.

Four cases with giant rugae of the stomach were classified by EUS into two types, one in which the thickness of the folds comprised the remarkable swelling of the mucosa; the other in which the thickness of the folds comprised the submucosal swelling. In the former, one of two cases was Menétrier's disease.

Figs. 4-15 and 4-16 are cases of colonic diseases. The thickness of the second and third layers characterized ulcerative colitis, and polypoid lesions in Cronkhite-Canada syndrome showed the hypoechoic swelling in the second layer.

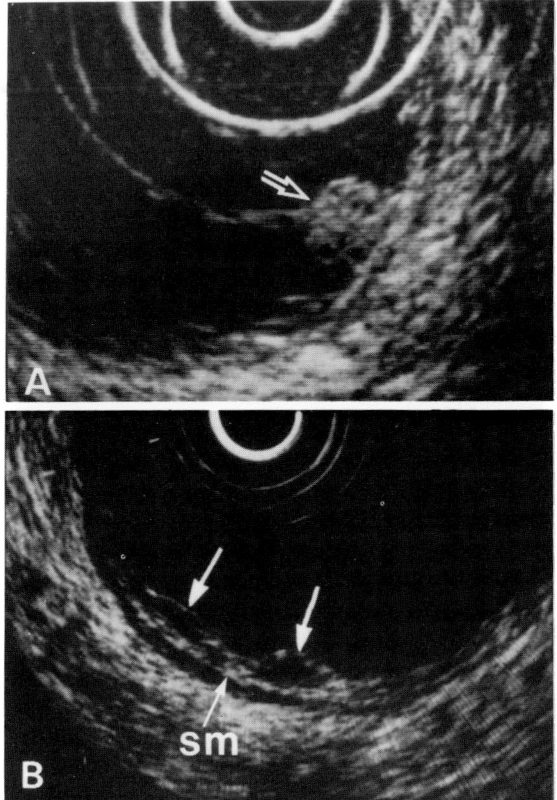

Fig. 4-16. Endoscopic ultrasonic findings of colon polyp. **A.** A case of adenoma. A polyp (black-white arrow) occurs in the first layer of the gastric wall. **B.** A case of Cronkhite-Canada syndrome. Polyps (arrows) exist in the second layer of the gastric wall and are visualized as hypoechoic lesions.

SUMMARY

EUS has many advantages over x-ray and other endoscopic procedures for detecting of lesions located in the gastrointestinal wall. In examining benign lesions of the gastrointestinal tract, EUS can accurately diagnose the submucosal tumor, including the genetic tissue, size and growth direction of the tumor, and the differential diagnosis between a malignant and benign tumor. This information contributes to the judgment of the possibility of various endoscopic therapies and determines the surgical adaptation for this lesion.

Peptic ulcer depth can be determined with EUS, and this technique seems to be able to predict the healing process and thus help in determining the best treatment of the ulcer. Furthermore, EUS also may be useful in the diagnosis of inflammatory disorders of the GI tract. The pathogenesis and healing process of AGML will be elucidated by EUS. In giant rugae of the stomach, a new diagnostic criteria, different from x-ray and other endoscopic procedures, may be established by this technique.

Detection in the colon by the present instrument is limited to the rectum and anal side of the sigmoid colon. However, a new view for the diagnosis of various inflammatory diseases in the colon will be achieved by the development of equipment exclusively for the colon.

In conclusion, the usefulness of endoscopic ultrasonography is highly appreciated in the diagnosis of benign lesions of the gastrointestinal tract, despite the fact that some problems still remain to be solved.

References

1. Aibe T, Fuji T, Okita K, Takemoto T: A fundamental study of normal layer structure of the gastrointestinal wall visualized by endoscopic ultrasonography. Scand J Gastroenterol 21 (Suppl 123): 6–15, 1986.
2. Takemoto T, Aibe T, Fuji T, Okita K: Endoscopic ultrasonography. In Classen M (ed): Endoscopy. Clinics in Gastroenterology, Vol. 15(2). W.B. Saunders Co., London, 1986, pp 305–319.
3. Yasuda K, Kiyota K, Mukai H, Nishimura K, Cho E, Kobayashi M, Yoshida S, Imaoka W, Fujimoto S, Nakajima M: Endoscopic ultrasonography (EUS) in the evaluation of endoscopic injection sclerotherapy (EIS) for esophago-gastric varices. Gastroenterol Endosc 28: 1788–1795, 1986 (with English abstract).

5

Malignant Lesions of the Gastrointestinal Tract

Kenjiro Yasuda, Masatsugu Nakajima, and Keiichi Kawai

The development of fiberoptic endoscopes has enabled us to diagnose easily malignant lesions in the gastrointestinal tract. Endoscopy allows us to see the surface of the gastrointestinal canal directly; however, the diagnosis of the invasion of malignant tumors is still based on the surface appearance of the lesion and the accuracy of the diagnosis depends on the experience of the endoscopist. Conventional ultrasonography (US) and computed tomography (CT) can provide us with three-dimensional images of the tumor. Under these circumstances, a new diagnostic method with which anyone can give a correct diagnosis of cancer invasion is expected.

Endoscopic ultrasonography (EUS), which combines the technique of endoscopy with that of ultrasonography, is a new method for intraluminal ultrasonographic scanning (5, 6, 12). We first used this technique in 1980 for the early diagnosis of pancreatic cancer (13, 14, 19). After we discovered that EUS could be used to delineate the gastrointestinal tract wall as a layered structure through water, we wanted to use EUS for diagnostic purposes in detecting gastrointestinal tract lesions (4, 9, 15).

EUS images of the gastrointestinal tract wall showed the wall to be a five-layered structure, in good correspondence with the histological layers (1, 2, 7). We confirmed this analysis by investigations in vivo and in vitro (12, 15). This five-layered structure formed the basis of our diagnosis of the gastrointestinal lesions. We have used echo-endoscopes with a 7.5-MHz or a 10.0-MHz sector-scan transducer to examine the GI tract lesions.

In EUS scanning, it is important to allow adequate distance between the lesion and the scanner, in order to fill this space with an echolucent substance. The deaerated water resolves this problem. There are two techniques for EUS scanning, one is the water-filling method, which allows observation of the gastric and colonic lesions; the other is the balloon-contact method, which allows observation of the esophageal and duodenal lesions. Often it is useful to combine these two methods. For such a situation, echo-endoscopes have a channel for pouring water into the digestive canal and can accommodate a rubber balloon around the transducer at the tip of the scope. In this chapter, we will discuss EUS images of malignant lesions in the digestive tract and the diagnostic effectiveness of EUS. Between April 1980 and December 1986, EUS was examined in 565 cases of gastrointestinal tract diseases (Table 5-1).

Table 5-1. Digestive tract diseases examined by EUS.

Esophagus			86
Cancer		20	
Early	7		
Advanced	13		
Submucosal tumorous lesion		30	
Submucosal tumor	25		
Extracompression	5		
Varices		34	
Others		2	
Stomach			400
Cancer		214	
Early	106		
Advanced	108		
Submucosal tumorous lesion		128	
Submucosal tumor	70		
Extracompression	58		
Ulcer		35	
Lymphoma		3	
Others		20	
Duodenum			9
Brunnerioma		2	
Submucosal tumorous lesion		4	
Submucosal tumor	4		
Ulcer		2	
Others		1	
Colon			70
Cancer		47	
Early	13		
Advanced	34		
Ulcerative Colitis		5	
Submucosal tumorous lesion		4	
Submucosal tumor	1		
Extracompression	3		
Others		14	
Total			565 cases

ENDOSCOPIC ULTRASONOGRAPHIC IMAGES OF THE NORMAL DIGESTIVE TRACT

ESOPHAGUS

Ultrasonograms of the esophagus can be obtained only by EUS. The image of the esophagus produced by the balloon-contact method or water-filling method of EUS is five-layered structure. However, the esophageal wall of the digestive tract has no scrosal layer. Without the serosal layer, the EUS image of the esophagus revealed the connective tissue in the mediastinum, considered to be the deepest layer. It was difficult to obtain an EUS image of the esophageal wall by the water-filling method because of the inability to retain water in the esophagus. The balloon-contact method should be used mainly for esophageal lesions. Using the balloon-contact method, the normal esophageal wall was observed as a five-layered structure. The first hyperechoic and second hypoechoic layers corresponded to the ultrasonogram of the mucosa (m) and that of the balloon itself. The third hyperechoic layer corre-

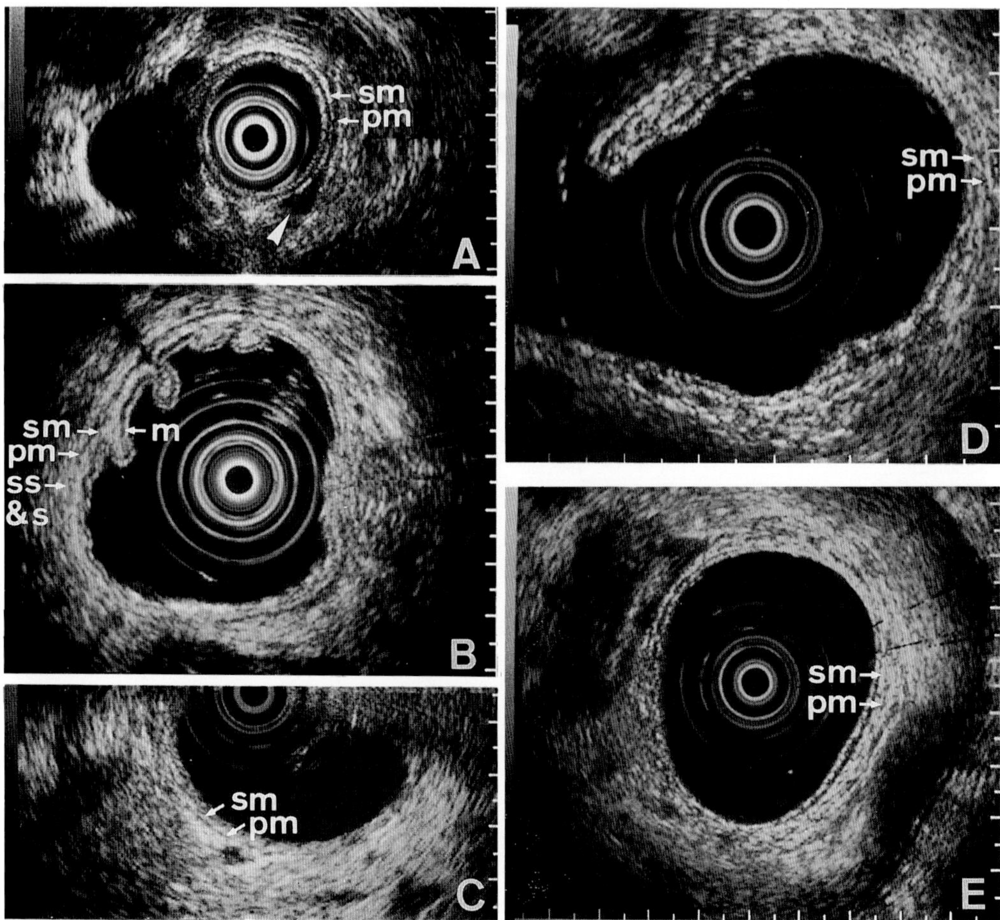

Fig. 5-1. EUS images of the normal digestive tract wall. m: mucosa; sm: submucosa; pm: proper muscle; s: serosa; ss: subserosa. **A.** Esophageal wall with a small submucosal tumor in the hypoechoic proper muscle layer (arrow) observed using the balloon-contact method. **B.** Gastric wall observed by an echo-endoscope with an improved 10.0-MHz sector-scan transducer, **C.** Duodenal bulbar wall observed, **D.** Sigmoid colon wall observed, and **E.** Rectal wall observed, all using the water-filling method.

sponds to the submucosal layer (sm), the fourth hyperechoic layer to the proper muscle (pm) layer, and the fifth hyperechoic layer corresponds to the connective tissue in the mediastinum. This analysis of the esophageal wall was confirmed by comparison with investigations in vivo and in vitro, yet it was difficult to determine the thickness of each layer. Fig. 5-1A shows the EUS image of the normal esophageal wall using the balloon-contact method with a small submucosal tumor in the proper muscle layer.

STOMACH

The gastric wall is the most suitable anatomical structure for employing the water-filling method of EUS. The EUS image of the gastric wall shows a five-layered structure and is in good correspondence with resected materials; the first hyperechoic and second hypoechoic layers correspond to the mucus, mucosa, and mucosal muscle (mm), the third hyperechoic layer corresponds to the submucosal layer, the fourth hypoechoic layer to the proper muscle layer, and the fifth hyperechoic layer corresponds to the subserosa (ss) and serosa (s). The thickness of each layer changed according to the degree of the expansion with water of the gastric wall, but the pattern of the layered structure was fixed. The fold of the stomach showed a characteristic image, differentiating the hyperplastic polyp or the protruded cancer from the normal wall structure.

Fig. 5-1B shows the EUS image of the normal gastric wall of the body of the stomach obtained by the water-filling method using an echo-endoscope with an improved 10.0 MHz sector scan transducer.

DUODENUM

Malignant lesions, except for lesions of the papilla of Vater, are rare in the duodenum (16). The duodenal canal is a narrow tract like the esophagus, in which it is difficult to store water for EUS scanning. Therefore, the balloon-contact method is more suitable for the duodenal EUS scanning. The bulbs of the duodenum have a layer of Brunner's glands, contained in the third hyperechoic layer. As a result, the third hyperechoic layer of the duodenum in the EUS image is thicker than that of other portions of the digestive tract. Occasionally, this hyperechoic layer divides into two layers: the layer of Brunner's glands and that of the submucosal layer in vivo. The other layers showed the same structure as the other portions of the digestive tract.

Fig. 5-1C shows the EUS image of the duodenal bulbs through water using an echo-endoscope with a 10.0 MHz sector scan transducer.

COLON

The echo-endoscopes that we have used were intended for the upper gastrointestinal examinations, hence, there are limitations to their use in colonoscopy. The echo-endoscope reaches the rectum and the lower sigmoid colon. The distinctive features of the colon are the existence of the haustra of the sigmoid colon and the lack of the serosa of the rectum. This anatomical feature creates serious problems in certain cases of colonic disease. That is, the lesions in the haustra, usually observed obliquely by EUS, were difficult to detect vertically in the EUS image. These two limitations prevent the full EUS study of the colon.

Fig. 5-1D shows the EUS image of the sigmoid colon, and Fig. 5-1E shows the EUS image of the rectal wall by the water-filling method using an echo-endoscope with a 7.5 MHz sector-scan transducer. The layered structure of the colon was delineated as a five-layered structure resembling the image of the gastric wall in vivo (3). In rare cases the fourth proper muscle layer of the colon wall could be observed dividing into two hypoechoic layers, following the direction of the muscle fibers.

ENDOSCOPIC ULTRASONOGRAPHIC IMAGES OF CANCER

Advanced cancer in the digestive tract appeared in the EUS images to be a hypoechoic irregular mass destroying at least the third submucosal layer (10, 12, 15). Cancers in the early stages showed mucosal changes with or without an irregularity of the third hyperechoic submucosal layer. A basic criteria for determining the depth of cancer invasion could be made from these images (Fig. 5-2).

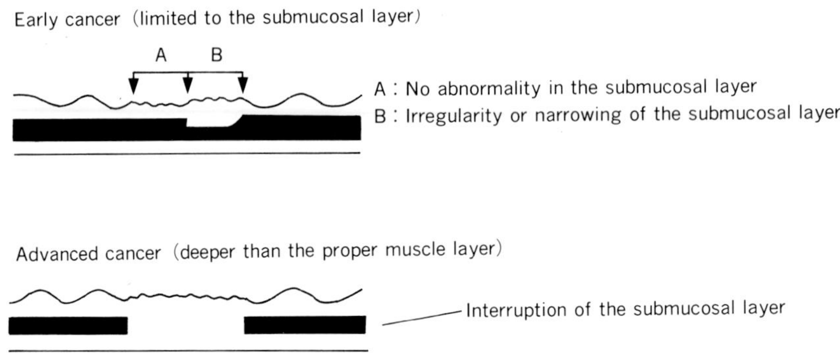

Fig. 5-2. EUS images of an early and advanced cancer of the stomach.

ESOPHAGEAL CANCER

In general, patients who are diagnosed as having esophageal cancer first come to the hospital complaining of dysphagia, the disturbance of the esophageal passage. As a result, esophageal cancers usually are diagnosed at an advanced stage. In some of these advanced cases, it is possible to examine only the upper end of the lesion with conventional endoscopy or echo-endoscopy because of the stenosis of the canal. Recently, a new instrument for examining esophageal lesions was developed, which has a short scope and allows direct viewing with a small-diameter tip. Fig. 5-3A shows an EUS image of an advanced cancer which was an inoperable case because of invasion of the cancer into the mediastinum. The echogram of tumor was observed as a hypoechoic irregular mass destroying the layered structure of the esophageal cancer limited to the proper muscle layer, and the hypoechoic tumor mass was detected on the hypoechoic proper muscle layer destroying the hyperechoic submucosal layer (Fig. 5-3B). Early esophageal cancer shows no abnormality in the submucosal layer (mucosal cancer). In submucosal cancer, the narrowing of the submucosal layer without interruption was detected, with or without detection of the ultrasonogram of the tumor itself. The accuracy rate was 78% in nine cases of esophageal cancer confirmed histologically by dividing the cases into mucosal, submucosal, proper muscle, and the deeper cancer.

In esophageal cancer, the diagnosis of the expansion to the extracanal region and the metastasis to the lymphnodes is still an unresolved problem despite recent progress of body-imaging diagnostics. Using EUS, we can determine cancer invasion to the mediastinal organs as well as to the metastic lymphnode of the paraesophageal regions. Figure 3C shows the paraesophageal metastic lymphnodes less than 5 mm in diameter. Thus, EUS images can provide information on areas beneath the mucosa and on the intramediastinal regions.

GASTRIC CANCER

Gastric cancer is a common disease among cancers of the digestive organs in Japan. As a result, diagnostic and therapeutic techniques have been developed using x-ray examination and fiberoptic endoscopes. However, diagnosis of the depth of the cancer invasion or the metastatic lymphnodes is difficult. Diagnosing the depth of gastric cancer invasion using EUS can be performed on the basis of the layered structure of the gastric wall (15, 18).

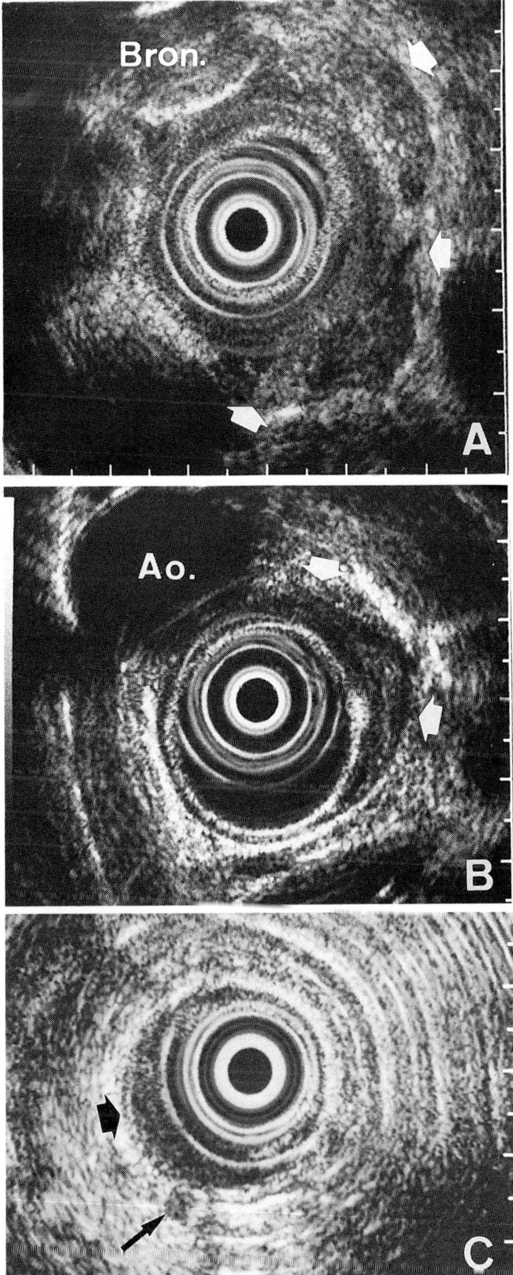

Fig. 5-3. EUS images of esophageal cancers. **A.** Advanced cancer invading the mediastinum with a hypo-echoic tumor mass showing an irregular inner echogram of the tumor destroying the layered structure of the normal esophageal wall. Bron.: bronchus. **B.** Advanced cancer limited to the proper muscle layer, showing a tumor echogram interrupting the submucosal layer. Ao.: aorta. **C.** Advanced cancer limited to the proper muscle layer with a metastatic lymphnode 5 mm in diameter (arrow).

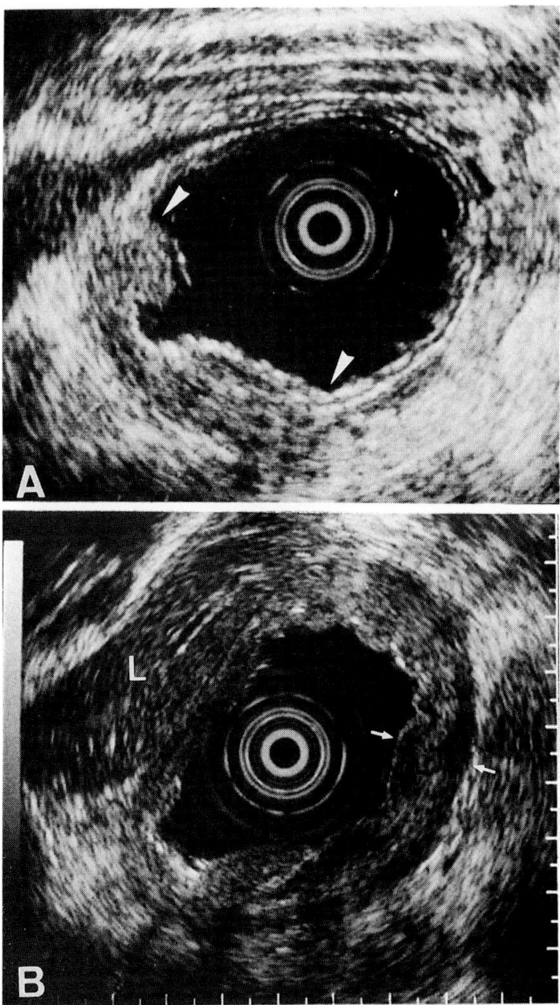

Fig. 5-4. EUS images of gastric cancers. **A.** Advanced cancer (Borrmann type III): A hypoechoic irregular tumor mass destroying the normal layered structure. **B.** Advanced cancer with a scirrhus invasion (Borrmann type IV), showing swelling and irregular gastric wall.

Advanced cancer was observed in the EUS image as the echogram of the tumor destroying the normal structure of the gastric wall. Fig. 5-4A shows the advanced gastric cancer (Borrmann type III) at the gastric angle. We observed a hypoechoic tumor mass with the ulcerative region and the destruction of the five layers around the tumor mass. Advanced gastric cancer with scirrhus invasion was observed to have its characteristic image, the swelling of the wall, and the diffuse destruction of the layered structure mainly in the submucosal and proper muscle layers (Fig. 5-4B).

On the other hand, as already mentioned, EUS images of early gastric cancer also were detected. Gastric cancer limited to the mucosa was observed only in the mucosal change and there was change under the submucosal layer. Fig. 5-5A shows the EUS image of an early protruded cancer of stomach (type IIa) limited to the mucosal layer. Early gastric cancer limited to the submucosa was observed in the EUS image as an irregularity of the submucosal layer with or without the echogram of the tumor. Fig. 5-5B shows an EUS image of early

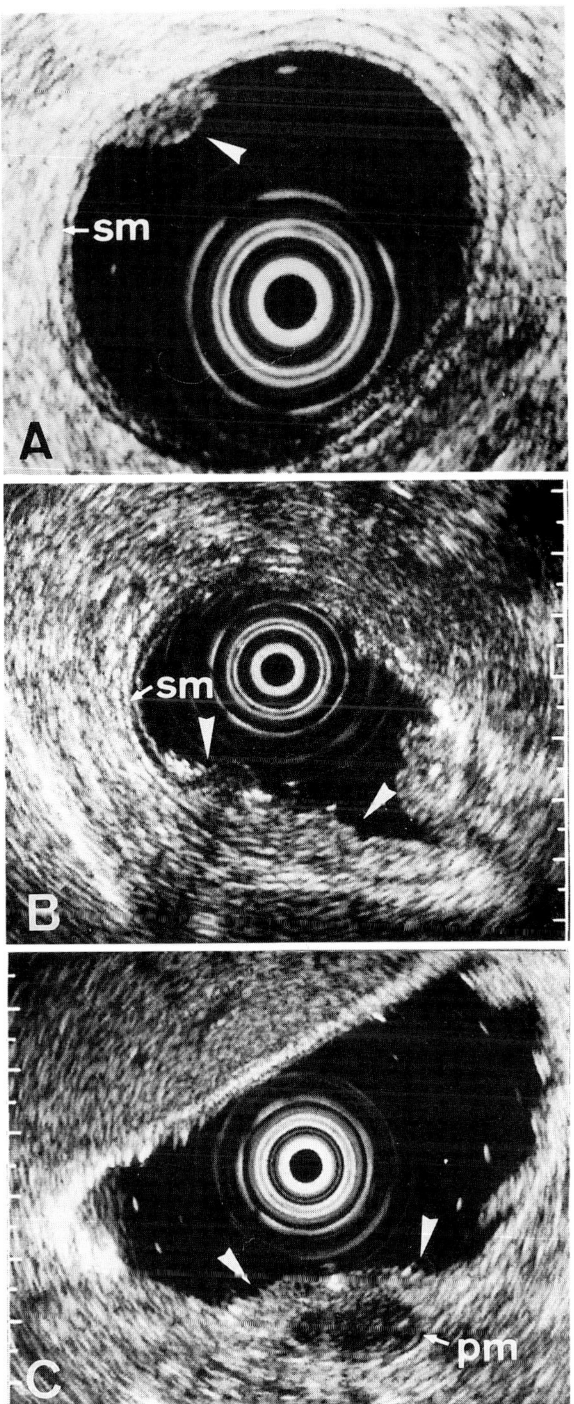

Fig. 5-5. EUS images of mucosa, submucosa, and proper muscle in each layer. **A.** Early protruded cancer (type IIa) limited to the mucosal layer, showing only a mucosal change in the first and second layers. **B.** Early cancer (type IIc) limited to the submucosal (sm) layer showing an irregular submucosal layer (arrow). **C.** Cancer limited to the proper muscle (pm) layer, showing an interruption of the third submucosal layer and no change in the fifth subserosal and serosal layers.

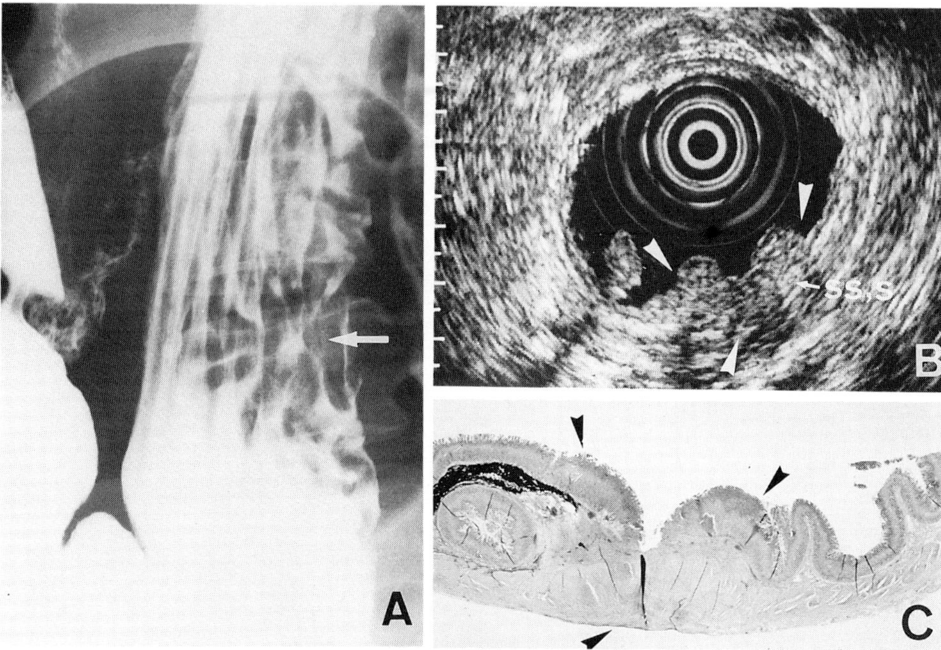

Fig. 5-6. Advanced cancer for which EUS was essential in determining the depth of the cancer invasion. **A.** X-ray examination showing malignant ulcerative changes in the body of the stomach. **B.** EUS image showing an ulcerative change with an abrupt interruption of the third submucosal layer and the fifth serosal layer. **C.** Histological finding revealed to be a cancer with an extraserosal invasion.

Table 5-2. Diagnostic accuracy rate for cancer invasion differentiated into early and advanced cancers (n = 144).

Histological diagnosis	EUS diagnosis		Total
	m·sm	pm $\leq$	
m·sm	62	9	71
pm $\leq$	5	66	71

accuracy rate: 90% (130/144).
m: mucosal; sm: submucosal; pm: proper muscle.

Table 5-3. Diagnostic accuracy rate for cancer invasion differentiated into mucosal, submucosal, proper muscle, and deeper-than-subserosal layers (n = 128).

Histological diagnosis/EUS diagnosis	m	sm	pm	ss $\leq$
m	30	9	3	2
sm	1	18	2	2
pm	0	2	7	3
ss $\leq$	0	0	1	47

Accuracy rate: 80% (102/128).
m: mucosal; sm: submucosal; pm: proper muscle; ss: deeper than subserosal.

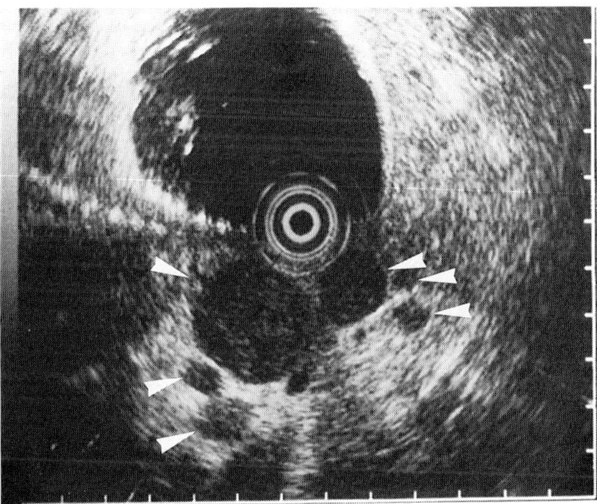

Fig. 5-7. EUS image of regional lymphnodes (arrow heads) observed in an advanced cancer.

Table 5-4. Accuracy rate of EUS in each histological type.

Type	Accuracy rate (%)	
Well differenciated adenocarcinoma	48/62	(77)
Moderately differenciated adenocarcinoma	12/17	(70)
Poorly differenciated adenocarcinoma	24/26	(92)
Mucinous adenocarcinoma	2/3	(67)
Signet-ring cell carcinoma	16/20	(80)
Total	102/128 (80)	

Table 5-5. Accuracy rate of EUS in types of cancer invasion.

Infiltration type	Accuracy rate (%)	
α	15/21	(71)
β	40/49	(82)
γ	42/52	(81)
Total	97/122 (80)	

Table 5-6. Accuracy rate of EUS in each position of the gastric lesion.

Position	Accuracy rate (%)	
Cardia	13/15	(87)
Body	46/59	(78)
Antrum	43/54	(80)
Total	102/128 (80)	

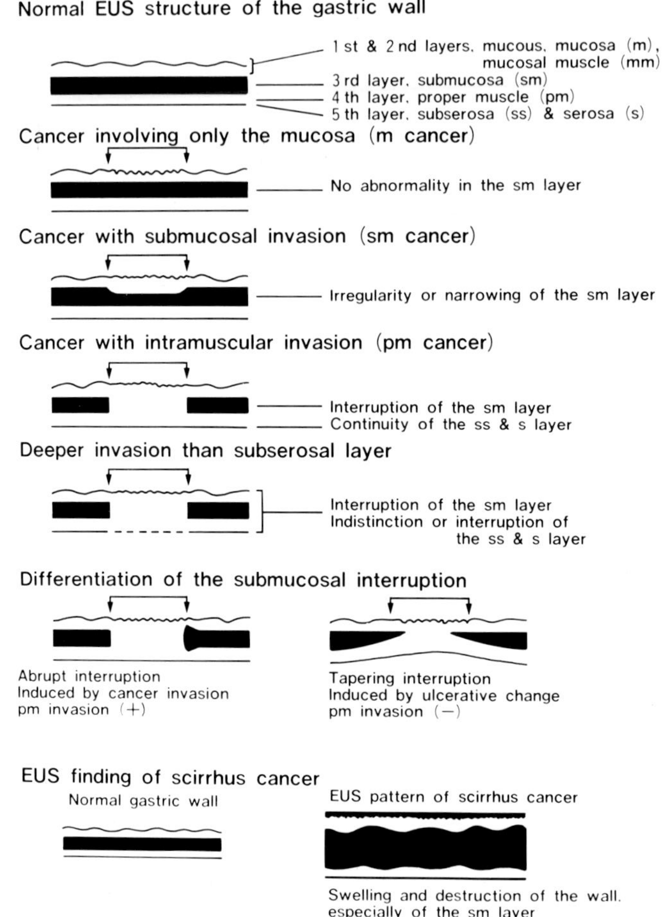

Fig. 5-8. Criteria for diagnosing the depth of cancer invasion using EUS.

gastric cancer (type IIc) limited to the submucosal layer. Gastric cancer limited to the proper muscle layer was observed in the EUS images as an interruption of the third submucosal layer with a clear echogram of the fifth layer (Fig. 5-5C). From these results, cancers were easily and exactly diagnosed by using EUS (Fig. 5-6). Fig. 5-7 shows criteria for understanding the depth of cancer expansion using EUS.

The diagnostic capability of EUS using these criteria in vivo is shown in Tables 5-2 and 5-3. In 144 cases of gastric cancer, 90% were accurately confirmed histologically by dividing the cases into early and advanced cancers. Furthermore, in 128 cases of gastric cancer, 80% were accurately confirmed histologically by dividing the cases into mucosal, submucosal, proper muscle, and deeper than subserosal cancer. There is no difference between the diagnostic capability of EUS in cell types, invasive types, and positions of the lesions (Tables 5-4 to 5-6). In the misdiagnosed cases using EUS, we judged most to be deeper in depth of cancer invasion than that of the histological finding. Unavoidable problems concern the diagnosis of the ulcerative change of the submucosal layer and the differential diagnosis of the cancer mass and fibrosis. The differentiation of cancerous and ulcerative interruptions of the submucosal layer are shown in Fig. 5-6. However, it is still difficult to differentiate cancer mass and fibrosis. The diagnosis of metastatic regional lymphnodes for cancer of the gastrointestinal tract is one of the most valuable uses of EUS (Fig. 5-8).

MALIGNANT LESIONS IN THE DUODENUM

Duodenal cancer, except for cancer of the papilla of Vater, is a rare disease. We have examined cancer of the papilla of Vater but have no experience examining duodenal cancer using EUS. In the diagnosis of duodenal cancer, the criteria of cancer invasion are the same as those of gastric cancer. However, in the lesions of the papilla of Vater, we have to discuss the EUS images on the invasion into the common bile duct, pancreas, and portal vein. Fig. 5-9 shows

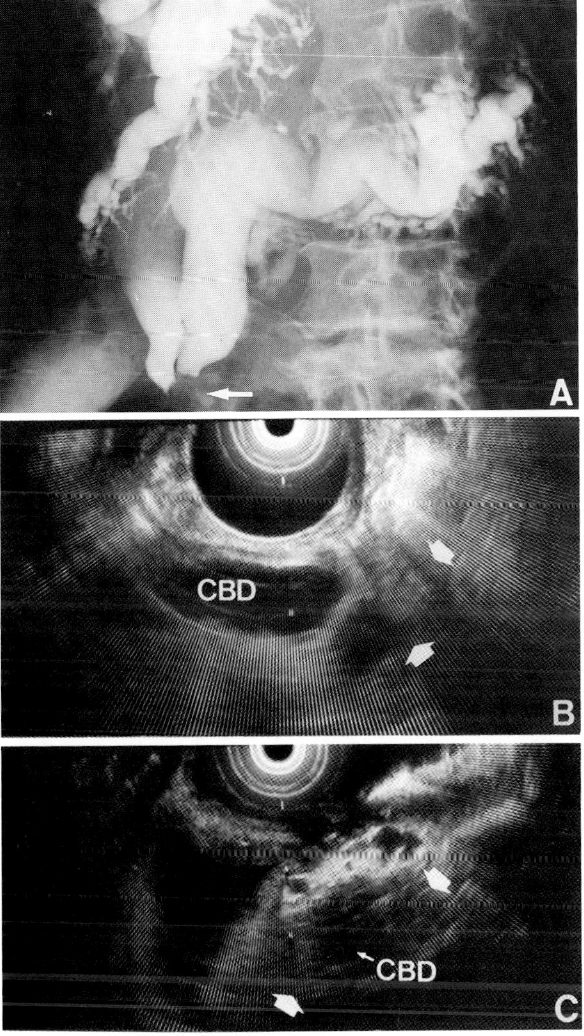

Fig. 5-9. EUS image of an early cancer of the papilla of Vater. CBD: common bile duct. **A.** ERCP finding showing the stenosis at the end of the pancreatobiliary junction (arrow). **B.** EUS image of the tumor obtained by the balloon-contact method from the duodenal second portion (arrows). **C** EUS image of the tumor by the balloon-contact method contacting the papilla of Vater (arrows).

EUS images of cancer of the papilla of Vater having a hypoechoic tumor with the echogram of the common bile duct (CBD).

COLON CANCER

EUS examination of the colon is limited to diseases of the rectum and lower colon because of the specification of echo-endoscopes. However, intraluminal scanning using EUS is one of its important diagnostic capabilities in examining intrapelvic diseases. Among other body-imaging diagnostics, only CT can provide tomographic images, but the capacity of CT is limited to large lesions.

EUS images of colon cancer provide the same information as that of gastric cancer through the water. The echogram of the cancer mass with a normal wall structure around the lesion can be detected. Fig. 5-10A shows an advanced sigmoid colon cancer reaching to the subserosa. The EUS image can provide exact information about the extraserosal lesion, but images of colon cancer usually are not especially clear because of residual stools. Fig. 5-10B shows early rectal cancer (a protruded lesion) in which the invasion was limited to the submucosal layer.

In 39 cases of rectosigmoidal cancer examined by EUS, the diagnostic accuracy rate was 77% (by dividing the cases into mucosal, submucosal, proper muscle, and deeper cancers)

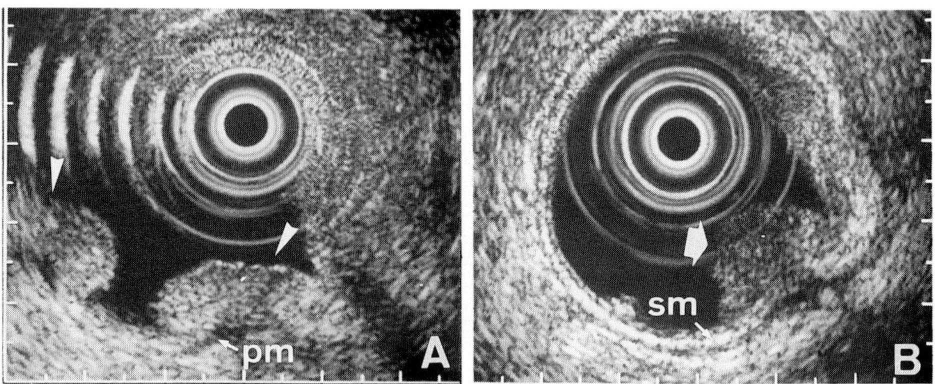

Fig. 5-10. EUS images of cancer of the colon. **A.** Advanced cancer limited to the subserosa. The tumor echogram destroying the normal wall structure was obtained by the water-filling method. pm: proper muscle. **B.** Early cancer limited to the submucosal layer (sm). The third submucosal layer beneath the tumor shows an irregular and narrow echogram.

Table 5-7. Diagnostic accuracy rate for colon cancer invasion differentiated into mucosal, submucosal, proper muscle, and deeper-than-subserosal layers (n = 39).

Histological diagnosis/EUS diagnosis	m	sm	pm	ss $\leqq$
m	3	0	1	0
sm	0	4	1	1
pm	0	0	5	4
ss $\leqq$	0	0	2	18

Accuracy rate: 77% (30/39).
m: mucosal; sm: submucosal; pm: proper muscle; ss: deeper than subserosal.

(Table 5-7). The accuracy rate in detecting gastric cancer is better because the haustra, the anatomical features of the colon, is not present in the gastric wall.

OTHER MALIGNANT LESIONS IN THE DIGESTIVE CANAL

MALIGNANT LYMPHOMA

According to EUS findings, malignant lymphomas of the gastrointestinal tract are delineated as characteristic features for each type of lymphoma (11). The ulcerative type of lymphoma showed a hypoechoic tumor mass beneath the ulcerative region, which is difficult to detect with an endoscope. Furthermore, the echogram of this tumor showed a diffuse hypoechoic mass compared with that of a cancer mass. This EUS image of a lymphoma mass is useful in evaluating the chemotherapy for the tumor. Fig. 5-11 shows the EUS image of a malignant lymphoma of the stomach before and after chemotherapy. It was clear that the hypoechoic tumor mass was reduced by the chemotherapy. Thus, EUS is useful as a monitor in determining the necessity of further treatment.

The infiltrating type of malignant lymphoma showed swelling of the layered structure like that in scirrhus cancer of the stomach.

MALIGNANT LESIONS IN SUBMUCOSAL TUMORS OF THE GASTROINTESTINAL TRACT WALL

The diagnosis of submucosal tumors is one of the most important functions of EUS (8, 17). The EUS image of a submucosal tumor provides information regarding its size and origin in the layered region of the submucosal tumor, and allows us to suggest a histological diagnosis. Submucosal tumors located in muscle layers such as the proper muscle layer can be diagnosed as leiomyoma or leiomyosarcoma. However, it is difficult to differentiate leiomyosarcoma from leiomyoma when using only EUS images without obtaining the true size of the tumor by EUS. Fig. 5-12 compares an EUS image of leiomyosarcoma with ulceration at the top of the submucosal tumor in the stomach with a leiomyoma of the same size.

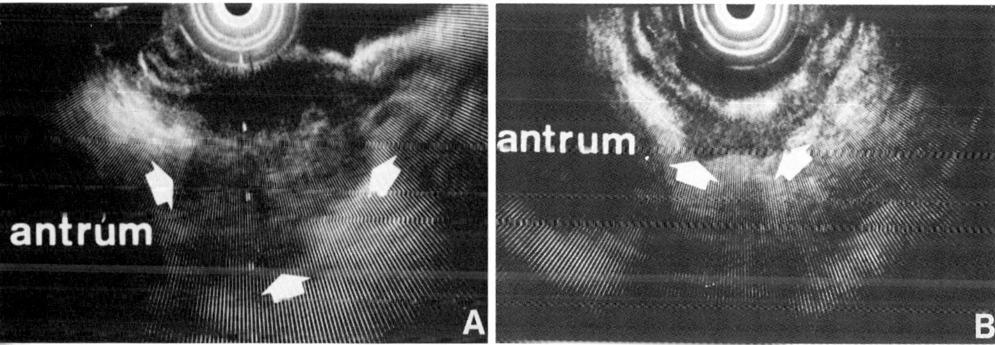

Fig. 5-11. EUS images of a malignant lymphoma before and after chemotherapy. antrum: gastric antrum.
A. Pretreatment observation of a hypoechoic large tumor mass, showing the intraperitoneal growth. **B.** Post-treatment observation of the tumor mass showing the tumor to be smaller, yet still detectable.

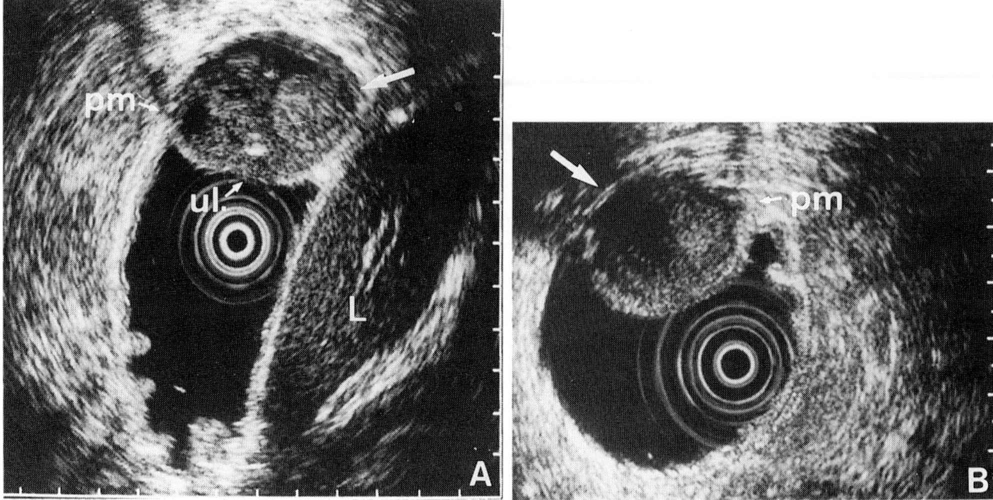

Fig. 5-12. EUS image of a leiomyosacrcoma compared with that of a leiomyoma. **A.** Leiomyosarcoma with an ulceration located in the proper muscle layer showing a hypoechoic irregular internal echogram. ul: ulceration; pm: proper muscle. **B.** Leiomyoma in the proper muscle layer difficult to differentiate from leiomyosarcoma, showing the same echogram as that of a leiomyoma.

CONCLUSIONS AND SUMMARY

EUS examination is a significant method for detecting malignant lesions in the gastrointestinal tract. Diagnosing the depth of cancer invasion correctly before surgery is one of the most important factors in determining the feasibility of the surgery as well as endoscopic treatment for early and advanced gastric cancer (12, 18).

By using EUS, we can correctly diagnose the depth of the cancer invasion. These three-dimensional images with an endoscopic view can provide us with information that has never been obtained by conventional body-imaging diagnostics. This diagnostic capacity is based on the analysis of the layered structure observed in the EUS image through water. However, the performance of echo-endoscopes is unsatisfactory for usual uses of endoscopy: they have no channel for biopsy or endoscopic treatments. Furthermore, the view of the endoscope is poor compared with conventional endoscopy. The tip length of the echo-endoscope is too long and the diameter of the endoscope is too large for usual uses.

EUS images of malignant lesions in vivo are useful not only in the diagnosis of lesion expansion but also as monitors of endoscopic laser treatment and chemotherapy. Thus, we have a new field of endoscopic diagnosis for malignant lesions in the gastrointestinal tract.

References

1. Aibe T, Fuji T, Okita K, Takemoto T: A fundamental study of normal layer structure of the gastrointestinal wall visualized by endoscopic ultrasonography. Scand J Gastroenterol 21 (Suppl 123): 6–15, 1986.
2. Bolondi L, Caletti G, Casanova P, Villanacci V, Grigioni W, Labo G: Problems and variations in the interpretation of the ultrasound feature of the normal upper and lower GI tract wall. Scand J Gastroenterol 21 (Suppl 123): 16–26, 1986.
3. Boscain M, Montori A: Transrectal ultrasonography: Interpretation of normal intestinal wall structure for the preoperative staging of rectal cancer. Scand J Gastroenterol 21 (Suppl 123) 87–98, 1986.

4. Caletti G, Bolondi L, Labò G: Anatomical aspects in ultrasonic endoscopy for the stomach. Scand J Gastroenterol 19 (Suppl 94): 34–42, 1984.

5. DiMagno EP, Buxton JL, Hattery RR, Wilson DA, Suarez JR, Green PS: Ultrasonic endoscope. Lancet 1: 629–631, 1980.

6. Hisanaga K, Hisanaga A, Nagata K, Ichie Y: High speed rotating scanner for transgastric sonography. AJR 135: 627–639, 1980.

7. Silverstein F, Kimmey M, Martin R, Haggitt R, Mack L, Moss A, Franklin D: Ultrasound and the intestinal wall: Experimental methods. Scand J Gastroenterol 21 (Suppl 123): 34–40, 1986.

8. Strohm WD, Classen M: Benign lesions of the upper GI tract by means of endoscopic ultrasonography. Scand J Gastroenterol 21 (Suppl 123) 41–46, 1986.

9. Tanaka Y, Yasuda K, Aibe T, Fuji T, Kawai K: Anatomical and pathological aspects in ultrasonic endoscopy for GI tract. Scand J Gastroenterol 19 (Suppl 94): 43–50, 1984.

10. Tio TL, Tytgat GNJ: Endoscopic ultrasonography of normal and pathologic upper gastrointestinal wall structure. Scand J Gastroenterol 21 (Suppl 123) 27–33, 1986.

11. Tio TL, Tytgat GNJ: Endoscopic ultrasonography in detection and staging of gastric non-Hodgkin lymphoma. Scand J Gastroenterol 21 (Suppl 123) 52–58, 1986.

12. Yasuda K, Kiyota K, Mukai H, Nishimura K, Cho E, Kobayashi M, Yoshida S, Imaoka W, Fujimoto S, Nakajima M, Tanaka Y, Kawai K: Clinical evaluation of endoscopic ultrasonography (EUS). Gastroenterol Endosc 26: 1911–1923, 1984.

13. Yasuda K, Tanaka Y, Fujimoto S, Nakajima M, Kawai K: Use of endoscopic ultrasonography (EUS) on the samall pancreatic cancer. Scand J Gastroenterol 19 (Suppl 102): 9–17, 1984.

14. Yasuda K, Mukai H, Yoshida S, Imaoka W, Fujimoto S, Nakajima M, Kawai K: Clinical evaluation of endoscopic ultrasonography (EUS) in the diagnosis of small pancreatic and biliary tumors. Gastroenterol Endosc 27: 943–954, 1985.

15. Yasuda K, Kiyota K, Mukai H, Nishimura K, Cho E, Kobayashi M, Yoshida S, Imaoka W, Fujimoto S, Nakajima M, Kawai K: Endoscopic ultrasonography (EUS) in the diagnosis of upper digestive tract disease. Determination of the depth of cancer invasion. Gastroenterol Endosc 28: 253–263, 1986.

16. Yasuda K, Nakajima M, Kawai K: Technical aspects of endoscopic ultrasonography of the biliary system. Scand J Gastroenterol 21 (Suppl 123): 143–150, 1986.

17. Yasuda K, Nakajima M, Kawai K: Endoscopic ultrasonography in the diagnosis of submucosal tumor of the upper digestive tract. Scand J Gastroenterol 21 (Suppl 123): 60–67, 1986.

18. Yasuda K, Kiyota K, Nakajima M, Kawai K: Fundamentals of endoscopic laser therapy (ELT) for G.I. tumors: New aspects with endoscopic ultrasonography (EUS). Endoscopy 19: 2–6, 1987.

19. Yasuda K, Mukai H, Fujimoto S, Nakajima M, Kawai K: The diagnosis of pancreatic cancer by endoscopic ultrasonography. Gastrointest Endosc 34: 1–8, 1988.

6

Pancreatic Cancer

Henryk Dancygier and Meinhard Classen

In the last few decades, the incidence of pancreatic cancer has increased steadily. Together with carcinoma of the lung, bowel, and breast, it is one of the leading causes of death in western countries today. Men are affected more often than women (1.5:1) and the peak incidence is between the ages of 60 to 70 years. The vast majority of pancreatic cancers are adenocarcinomas arising from the duct epithelium. Most are localized in the head of the pancreas (60%), followed by the body (13%) and the tail (5%). Twenty-one percent originate at multiple sites, mostly the body and tail (7).

Although many patients with pancreatic cancer undergo laparotomy, at diagnosis the tumor is confined to the pancreas in only 10 to 15% of cases, and resection aimed at cure is performed in only about 10%. The overall survival rate is less than 5% (6). The prognosis of ampullary carcinomas is much better since these tumors cause relatively early clinical signs, such as jaundice and pain: approximately every third patient survives five years after operation (1).

Laboratory findings such as enzyme abnormalities, serological tumor markers, and pancreatic function tests are not helpful in the early detection of pancreatic cancer. Ultrasonography is a valuable initial screening procedure but tumors smaller than 2 cm are rarely found, and carcinomas in the body and tail are difficult to recognize. CT scanning allows a better definition of the pancreatic body and tail than sonography, but false-negative results occur in up to 15% of cases. Selective angiography undoubtedly has its value in preoperative assessment of vessel displacement and vessel patency, but obviously it cannot be employed on a large scale in the search of pancreatic cancer. Endoscopic retrograde cholangiopancreatography (ERCP) has a diagnostic accuracy in pancreatic cancer of about 80%, but the differentiation between carcinoma and chronic pancreatitis often is difficult. Nuclear magnetic resonance imaging (MRI) has not yet gained practical importance in the diagnosis of pancreatic cancer, and radionuclide pancreatic scintigraphy is of only limited value.

These data highlight the need for a method that allows for a better visualization of the entire pancreatic region. With the development of small sonographic probes attached to the tip of flexible endoscopes we have come one step closer to this goal. Modern endosonographic scopes work with high ultrasound frequencies (7.5 to 10 MHz) and therefore provide an excellent detail resolution that enables us to delineate the entire pancreas with a hitherto unknown precision.

ENDOSONOGRAPHIC EXAMINATION OF THE PANCREAS

After premedication the patient is examined in the left lateral decubitus position. The tip of the instrument is introduced into the second portion of the duodenum and is then slowly pulled back, rotating the transducer around its long axis. In the duodenum and the prepyloric antrum ultrasonic beam transmission is optimized by inflating a small balloon with water around the sonographic probe. From these positions the peripapillary region as well as the head of the pancreas are best visualized. The instrument is then pulled back into the body and fundus of the stomach, which are filled with 200 to 300 ml of deaerated water. Again, rotation around the long axis as well as flexion of the tip of the instrument are important maneuvers in visualizing the pancreatic body and tail. In addition to movements of the instrument during this phase of the investigation, the patient should be turned on his back and/or to the prone position.

ENDOSONOGRAPHIC APPEARANCE OF THE NORMAL PANCREAS

The splenic artery and vein and the portal vein are the guiding topographical structures of the pancreatic region. The normal pancreas is characterized by a homogeneous dense echopattern disrupted only by the hypoechoic structures that belong to the common bile duct, Wirsung's duct, and splenic vessels. The outer contours of the organ are sharply delineated, but sometimes the lobulated architecture may be evident, which must not be confused with chronic pancreatitis. The main pancreatic duct measures between 1 and 2 mm in diameter, has a smooth outer margin, and may be lined by two slim echogenic bands. It is easily demonstrated in the body and tail. Its visualization in the head of the pancreas is more difficult.

ENDOSONOGRAPHIC ASPECT OF PANCREATIC CANCER

In most cases, pancreatic cancer presents as a circumscribed echo-poor lesion with an uneven, irregular structural pattern and with polycyclic and sometimes flamelike outer margins (Figs. 6-1 to 6-3). Echogenic tumors with an echo-free outer rim also are characteristic, albeit rare (Figs. 6-4 and 6-5). Most cases of pancreatic cancer presented to the physician already have grown beyond the outer margins of the organ. Because of their size they often are difficult to delineate on endosonography. As a rule, it may be stated that small lesions (< 2 cm) within a normal organ are better seen endosonographically than large alterations. Isolated cystic lesions smaller than 1 cm in diameter in a normal organ without any signs of chronic pancreatitis should be suspected to be small, centrally-necrotic carcinomas until proved otherwise (Fig. 6-6). Each investigation for pancreatic cancer also should include a search for metastatic peripancreatic and periceliac lymphnodes and metastases in the left liver lobe (Fig. 6-7).

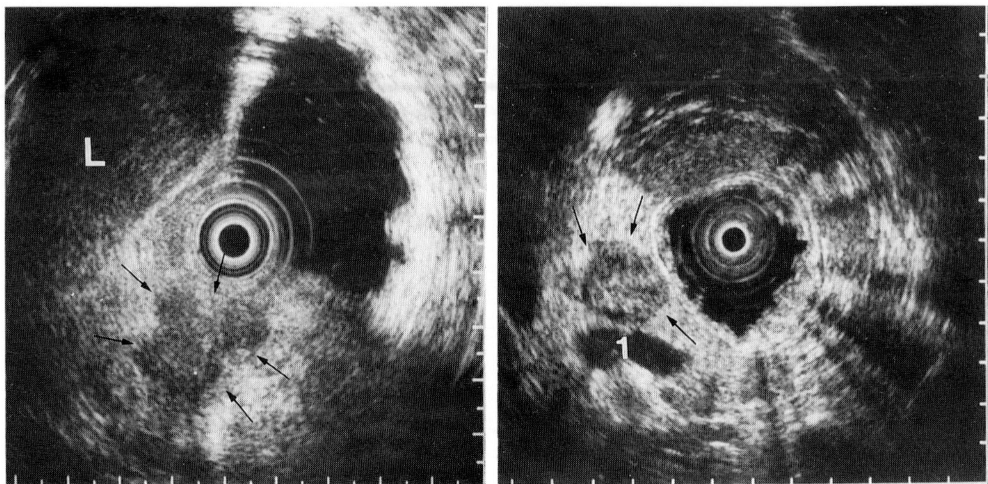

Fig. 6-1.   **Fig. 6-2.**

Fig. 6-1.   Pancreatic carcinoma (arrows).   Note echo-poor structure and polycyclic outer margin.   L: liver.

Fig. 6-2.   Pancreatic carcinoma (arrows).   Mixed echo-pattern, relatively sharp margin.   1: splenic vein.

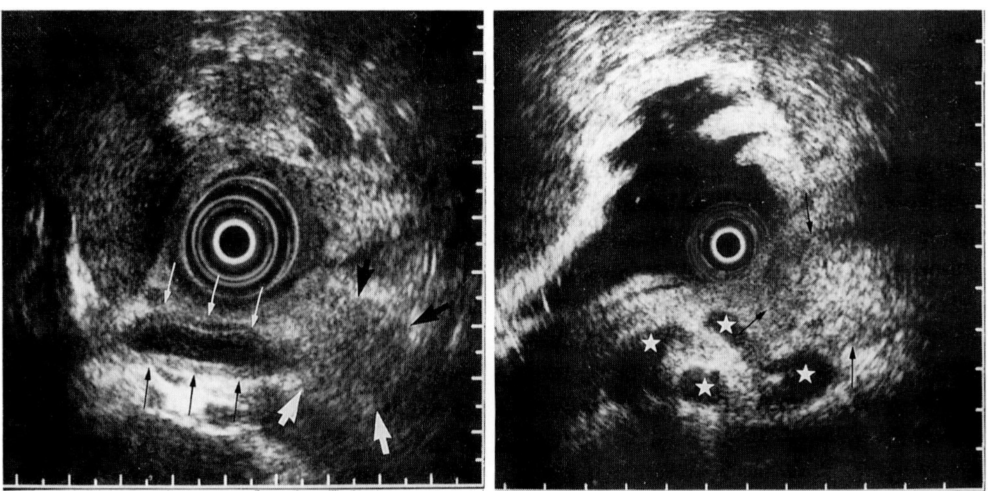

Fig. 6-3.   **Fig. 6-4.**

Fig. 6-3.   Echo-poor papillary tumor (thick arrows) leading to stenosis of the common bile duct (slim arrows).   Note clear demonstration of the wall of the common bile duct.

Fig. 6-4.   Tumor in the pancreatic tail (arrows) with an echogenic center and an echo-poor outer rim. Asterisks denote pancreatic and splenic vessels.

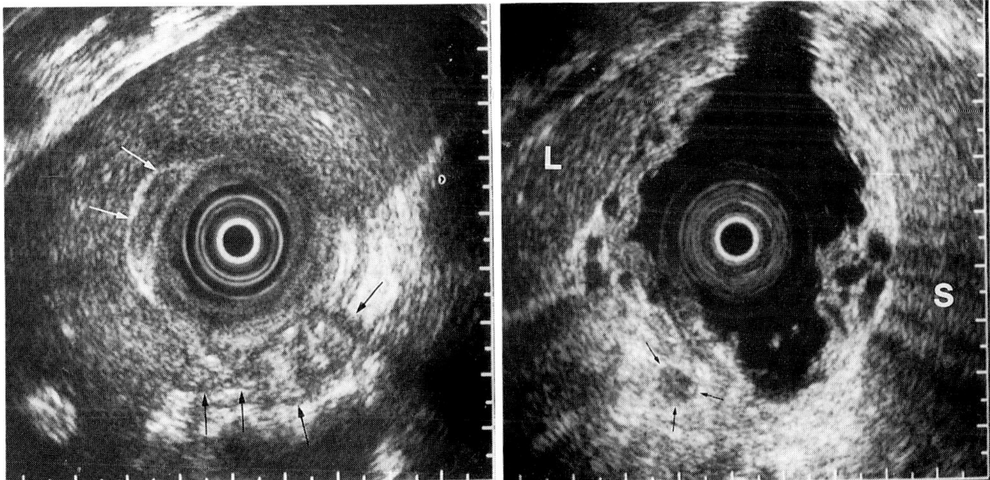

Fig. 6-5.   Fig. 6-6.

Fig. 6-5. Pancreatic cancer. Mixed central echo-pattern and echo-poor outer rim (black arrows). Contracted gallbladder (white arrows).

Fig. 6-6. Echo-poor lesion (arrows) in pancreatic body. Such lesions should be operated on. L: liver; S: spleen.

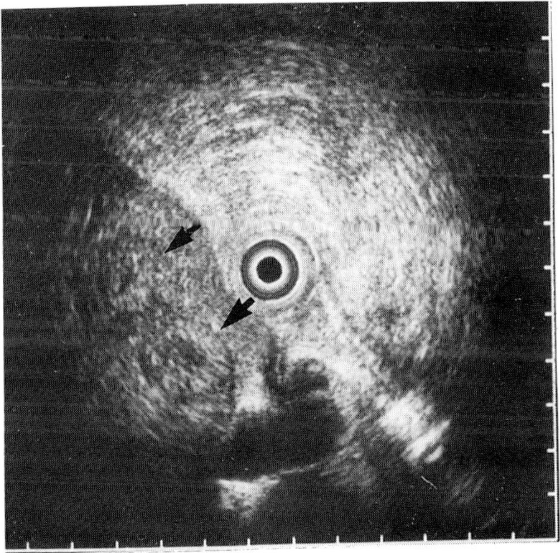

Fig. 6-7. Two target-type metastases in left liver lobe (arrows).

ENDOSONOGRAPHIC DIFFERENTIAL DIAGNOSIS OF PANCREATIC CANCER

The main difficulty in differential diagnosis of pancreatic cancer is the distinction between malignant lesions and benign alterations seen in chronic pancreatitis. This latter condition usually involves large portions of the pancreas and has an irregular structural appearance (Figs.

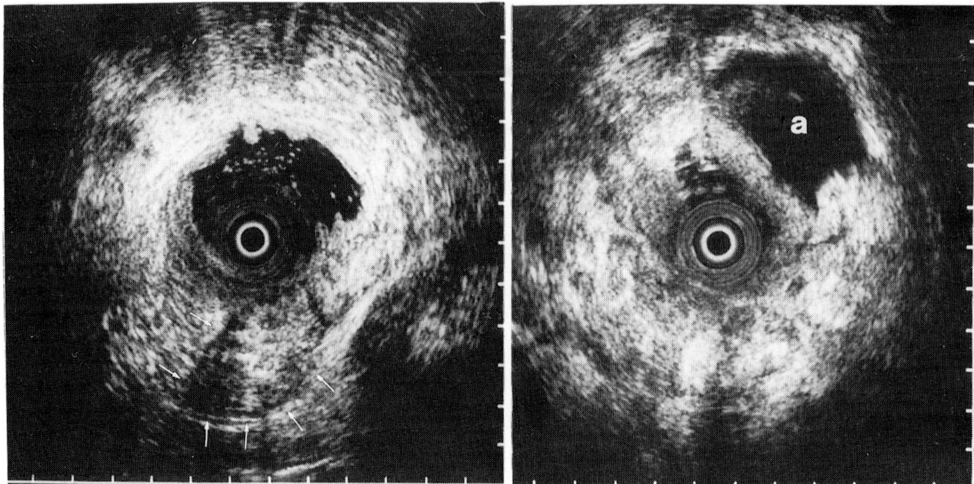

Fig. 6-8.   Fig. 6-9.

Fig. 6-8.   Chronic pancreatitis involving nearly the entire pancreas (arrows).

Fig. 6-9.   Chronic pancreatitis. Irregular reflex pattern with bright echoes. The entire organ is involved (lower half of picture). a: ascites.

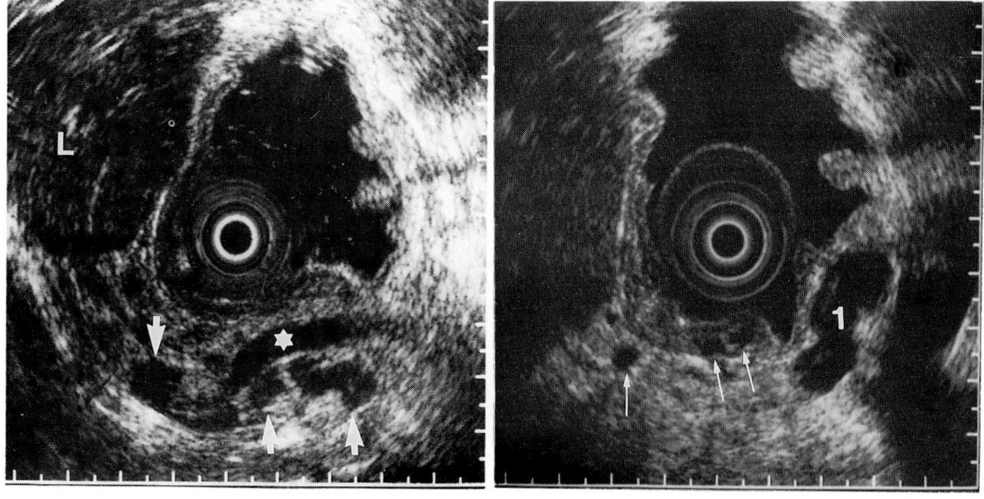

Fig. 6-10.   Fig. 6-11.

Fig. 6-10.   Pseudocysts (arrows). Dilated, but smoothly outlined pancreatic duct (asterisk). L: liver.

Fig. 6-11.   Dilated paragastric and intramural veins in portal hypertension (arrows). 1: dilated splenic vein.

6-8 and 6-9).   The demonstration of broad reflexes with associated shadows caused by parenchymal or ductal calcifications along with microcysts strongly favor the diagnosis of chronic pancreatitis.   However, it often remains impossible to recognize a carcinomatous lesion in a chronic inflammatory surrounding.   Benign (pseudo)cysts are sharply demarcated and often multiple (Fig. 6-10).   Since pseudocysts contain necrotic tissue and cellular debris, their echopattern may be mixed or may display an increased echogenicity (3), thus making it difficult to differentiate a carcinoma from a cystadenoma.   A cystadenoma, as well as its malignant counterpart, the cystadenocarcinoma, is characterized by a septated appearance. Metast   lesions to the pancreas caused by malignant lymphoma and enlarged paragastric lymphnodes in gastric cancer also must be kept in mind when echo-poor lesions are found. Cross-sectioned dilated gastric veins in portal hypertension present as small, round, echo-free lesions (Fig. 6-11). These alterations do not pose diagnostic difficulties because of their sharp margins, their position adjacent to the gastric wall, their typical "lined up" appearance, and the concomitant finding of an enlarged splenic vein.

DIAGNOSTIC EFFICIENCY OF ENDOSONOGRAPHY IN PANCREATIC CANCER

The number of clinical trials in which endosonography has been tested in the diagnosis of pancreatic cancer is limited. In 118 patients examined by endosonography, Yasuda et al. (9) found pancreatic carcinoma in 13 cases. Nine of these tumors were larger than 3 cm in diameter and one had a diameter of 2.5 cm, whereas the remaining 3 cases were of tumors smaller than 2 cm in diameter. All pancreatic cancers were echo-poor. In 10 of these 13 cases, ERCP, CT, and angiography were performed in addition to conventional and endoscopic ultrasound. The positive finding rate of endosonography reported by the authors was 100%, whereas conventional ultrasound resulted in a 40% rate, ERCP was 80%, CT was 70%, and angiography was 80%. All three tumors smaller than 2 cm did not show metastases and were resected. From these studies, the authors conclude that, compared with ERCP, CT, angiography, and conventional ultrasound, "endosonography is the most useful method for the demonstration of small pancreatic carcinomas of less than 20 mm in size" (9). In another study (8) aimed at investigating the sensitivity and specificity of endosonography compared with conventional morphological methods in the diagnosis of pancreatic cancer, Strohm et al. examined 34 patients with painless jaundice. Endosonography was performed after conventional ultrasound. Three tumors of Vater's papilla were detected by endosonography, whereas conventional ultrasound detected only one. Ten pancreatic cancers with an average size of 2.8 cm in diameter were diagnosed by endosonography. According to the authors, endosonography permitted a more precise description of outer tumor margins and of the inner echo-structure compared with conventional ultrasound so that in addition to the demonstration of a pathological lesion, endosonographic criteria allowed a better discrimination between benign and malignant alterations. Six of their cases were echo-poor, two echo-dense, and two showed a mixed reflex pattern. It was remarkable that four malignant tumors showed smooth outer contours.

Both studies are laudable efforts to assess objectively the diagnostic efficiency of endosonography in the diagnosis of pancreatic cancer. The endosonographic demonstration of a large tumor that already has been visualized by other methods is of course of no prognostic advantage to the patient. An interesting starting point for future prospective studies that must aim at the endosonographic diagnosis of potentially curable resectable tumors is the ability of the method to demonstrate small tumors that escape delineation with conventional methods (2, 4). However, owing to the natural course of pancreatic carcinoma, a systematic early detection of this neoplasia with endoscopic ultrasound is not to be expected. In this case, too, endosonography is to be viewed as a complementary method (5).

It is hoped that with further technical improvements and more experience with this method, endosonography will find a definite place in the early examination of a patient with suspected pancreatic cancer, so that the cure rate will increase.

References

1. Awari OE, Van Heerden JA, Adson MA, Baggenstoss AH: Radical pancreatoduodenectomy for cancer of the papilla of Vater. Arch Surg 112: 451-456, 1977.
2. Dancygier H: Endoskopische Sonographie—ein diagnostischer Fortschritt im oberen Verdauungstrakt? Leber Magen Darm 16: 114-120, 1986.
3. Dancygier H, Classen M: Endoscopic diagnosis of benign pancreatic and biliary lesions. Scan J Gastroenterol 21 (Suppl 123): 119-122, 1986.
4. Dancygier H, Classen M: Endoskopische Sonographie des oberen Verdauungstraktes. Med Klin 81: 92-96, 1986.
5. Dancygier H, Classen M: Endoscopic sonography of pancreatic cancer. Front Gastrointest Res 12: 195-207, 1986.
6. Gudjonsson B, Livstone EM, Spiro HM: Cancer of the pancreas. Diagnostic accuracy and survival statistics. Cancer 42: 2492-2506, 1978.
7. Russel RCG: Carcinoma of the pancreas and ampulla of vater. In Misiewicz JJ, Pounder RE, Venables CW (eds): Diseases of the Gut and Pancreas. Blackwell Scientific Publications, Oxford, 1987, p 549.
8. Strohm WD, Kurtz W, Hagenmüller F, et al.: Diagnostic efficacy of endoscopic ultrasound tomography in pancreatic cancer and cholestasis. Scan J Gastroenterol 19 (Suppl 102): 18-23, 1985.
9. Yasuda K, Tanaka Y, Fujimoto S, et al.: Use of endoscopic ultrasonography in small pancreatic cancer. Scan J Gastroenterol 19 (Suppl 102): 9-17, 1984.

7
Chronic Pancreatitis

Saburo Nakazawa, Yoshiki Hayashi, Yasuo Naitoh, Eizo Kimoto, Kenji Yamao, Keiichi Morita, and Kazuo Inui

Ultrasonography (US) is an important tool in diagnosing pancreatic disease because of its convenience and low cost (3). However, factors such as bowel gas and fatty abdominal wall restrict its clinical use. The higher frequency transducer is limited in conventional ultrasonography because of its poor penetration of the sound beam. Endoscopic ultrasonography (EUS) has now been developed to overcome these problems and improve the quality of pancreatic sonograms (2, 7). EUS already has proved useful in diagnosing pancreatic cancer, especially small cancers (6, 10). Recently, this technique has been found to be useful in other gastrointestinal tract diseases (8, 9) as well as the gallbladder (5). Since current diagnostic modalities often are inconclusive when diagnosing chronic pancreatitis, EUS may prove more appropriate. The advantages and disadvantages of using EUS to detect chronic pancreatitis are discussed in this chapter.

THE PANCREATIC ULTRASONOGRAPHIC EXAMINATION

We used EUS (GF-UM2) on 100 patients who we examined either from the stomach or the second portion of the duodenum. The entire pancreas, including the head, body, tail, and main pancreatic duct (MPD), was visualized. By using conventional ultrasound (Toshiba SSA-90A), on the other hand, we achieved a 60% visualization rate for the head, 100% for the body, 25% for the tail, and 61% for the MPD in the same patients (Table 7-1). This result agrees with other reports of pancreatic imaging using extracorporeal ultrasonic examination (1, 4). Ultrasonic imaging of the entire pancreas is possible with EUS because the transducer is introduced close to the pancreas. However, the movement of the transducer is somewhat

Table 7-1. Visualization of pancreas parts by US and EUS in 100 cases*.

	Head (%)[†]	Body (%)	Tail (%)	MPD (%)
US	60	100	25	61
EUS	100	100	100	100

US: Toshiba SSA-90A (3.75 MHz); EUS: Olympus GF-UM2 (7.5 MHz, 10 MHz).
*From May to December 1986.
[†]Percentage of cases in which the part was visible.
MPD: main pancreatic duct.

restricted in EUS because the scanning requires contact with the wall of the gastrointestinal tract (that is, the descending part of the duodenum and the corpus of the stomach).

DIAGNOSIS OF CHRONIC PANCREATITIS

From January 1982 to September 1986, we performed EUS in 150 patients with suspected or confirmed pancreatic disease, including 48 cases of chronic pancreatitis (22 cases of calcified and 26 noncalcified) diagnosed by conventional ultrasound, endoscopic retrograde cholangio-

Table 7-2. Characteristic findings in chronic pancreatitis obtained by US, EUS, CT, and ERP.

Findings	US (N = 48)	EUS (N = 48)	CT (N = 47)	ERP (N = 46)
Lithiasis	12	19	20	13
	(AS + SE) 8	(AS + SE) 19		(XP pos) 7
Duct dilatation				
MPD	23	33	24	27
branch (cystic, irregular)	0	25	0	40
MPD obstruction	—	4(?)	—	13
MPD stenosis	1	1	—	13
Mass	7	6	4	—
Cyst				
more than 20 mm	6	7	9	2
less than 20 mm	2	8	2	11
Heterogenous parenchyma	0	32	0	—

MPD: main pancreatic duct; AS: acoustic shadow; SE: strong echo; XP pos: radio-opaque on plain x-ray; ERP: endoscopic retrograde pancreatography.
ERP did not succeed in two cases: one had partial gastrectomy (Billroth II), in the other, insertion of cannula was not successful.

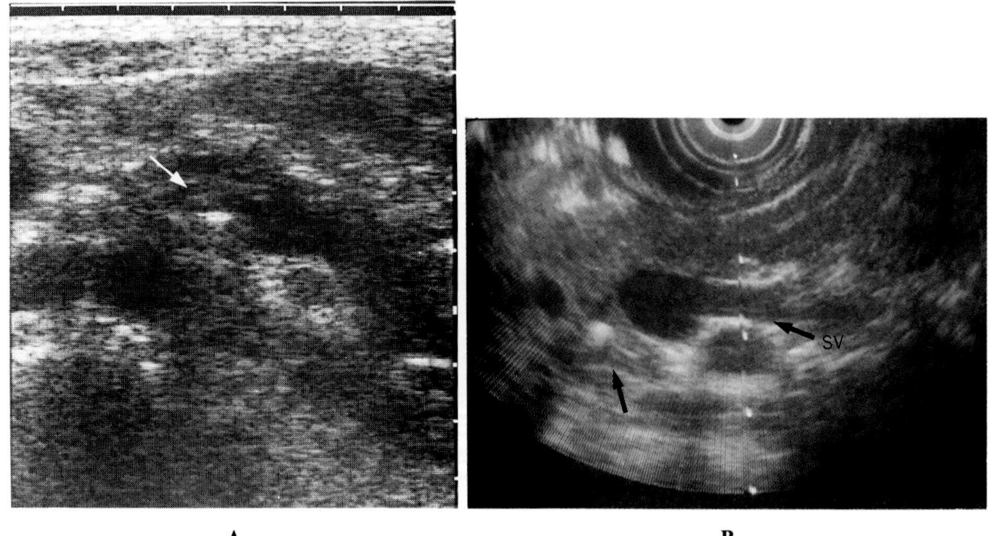

A   B

Fig. 7-1. **A:** A solitary SE (strong echo) without AS (acoustic shadow) is demonstrated by conventional US (arrow). **B:** By EUS, SE and AS are clearly seen (arrow). SV: splenic vein.

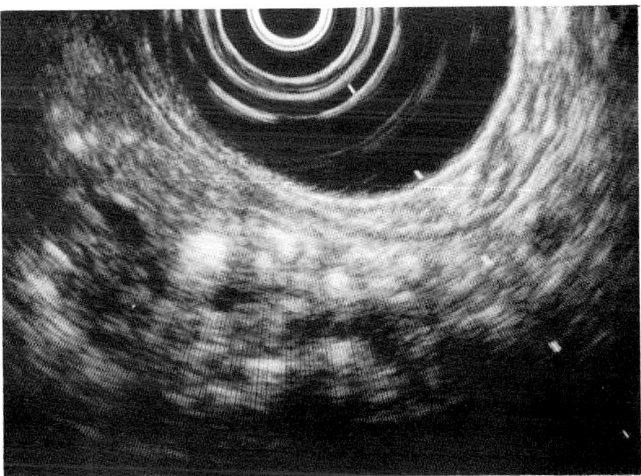

Fig. 7-2. Pancreatolith (multiple). Pancreatic duct and parenchyma are obscured by many stones.

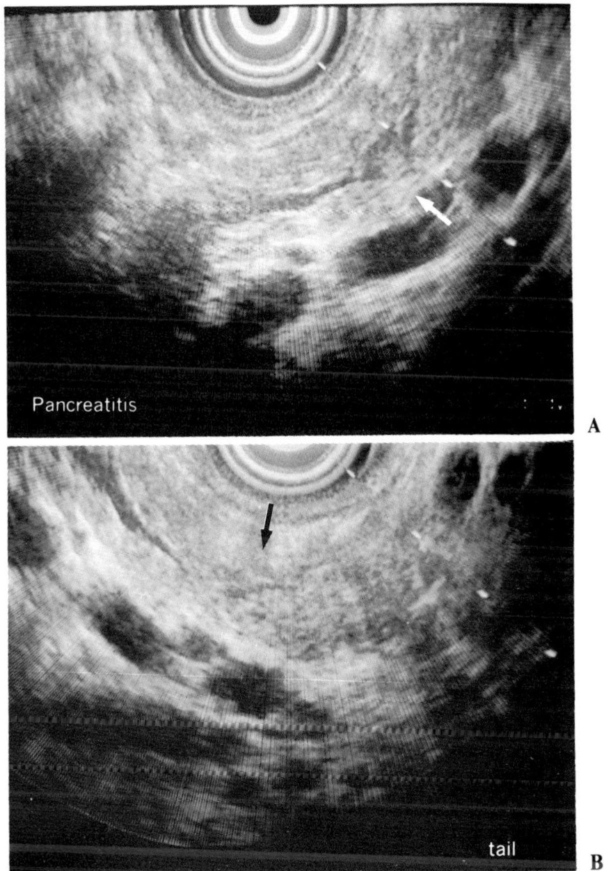

Fig. 7 3. Dilated main pancreatic duct and branches (body). **B:** Dilated pancreatic branches (tail).

pancreatography (ERCP), and computed tomography (CT). Each characteristic finding by EUS in these 48 patients with chronic pancreatitis was compared favorably with the other diagnostic techniques (Table 7-2). The detectability of abnormal findings by EUS is superior to all the other types of diagnostic imaging techniques owing to EUS's ability to visualize the entire pancreas with a high-resolution image.

PANCREATOLITH

Pancreatoliths appear ultrasonographically as strong echoes (SEs) and acoustic shadows (ASs), although some SEs will appear in exceptional cases without ASs. Pancreatoliths were detected in 12 cases (55%) by US, 19 (86%) by EUS, 20 (91%) by CT, and 13 (59%) by ERCP. In four cases, SE with an ill-defined acoustic shadow was demonstrated by ultrasound, which was clearly recognized as a pancreatolith by EUS (Fig. 7-1). Acoustic shadowing occurs more frequently with EUS than US, probably because the sound beam attenuates more easily. However, when there are multiple pancreatoliths, SEs prevent clear images of the pancreatic duct and parenchyma, just as they do in conventional ultrasound (Fig. 7-2). In such cases, CT is superior to other diagnostic imaging methods to demonstrate the size and distribution of the stones. Nevertheless, EUS differentiates protein plugs from pancreatoliths when isolated intraductal lesions are visualized on ERCP, whereas high-contrast radiograms do not.

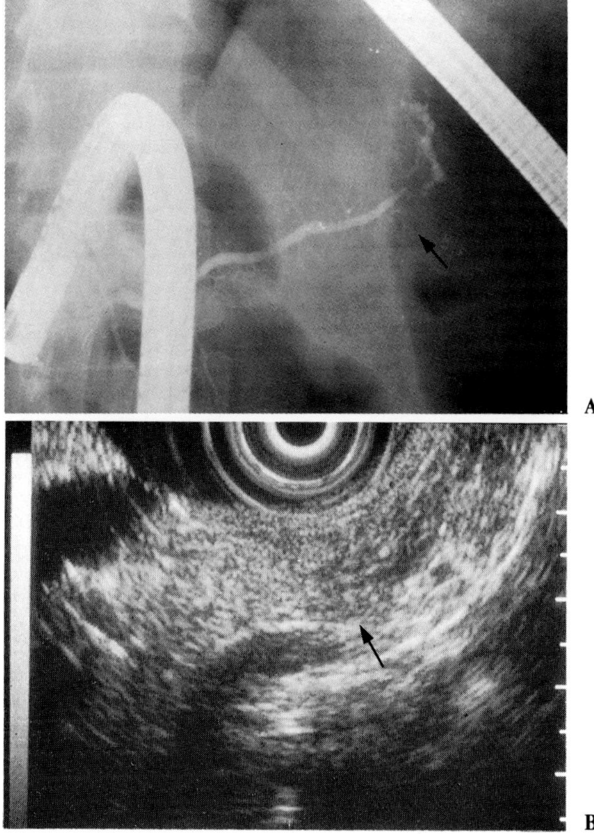

Fig. 7-4. A: Localized stenosis of the main pancreatic duct (tail) as shown by ERCP. **B:** With EUS, no tumor can be seen at the stenosis of the dilated pancreatic duct showing with heterogenous echo-pattern of the parenchyma caudal to the stenosis.

DILATATION OF PANCREATIC DUCTS

Main Pancreatic Duct
A dilated MPD was identified in 23 cases (48%) by US, 33 (69%) by EUS, 24 (50%) by CT, and 27 (56%) by ERCP. Assessment of the pancreatic ductal system is best done by ERCP because it provides the clearest images and yields the greatest amount of information about the ductal system in cases of pancreatitis. By EUS, the MPD was demonstrated more frequently and clearly than US or CT (Fig. 7-3). Even if ERCP cannot be performed or pancreatic ductal stenosis prevents opacification of the distal duct, EUS usually can image the main duct and disclose the changes in the ductal wall clearly. In eight of 13 cases in which the distal ductal system was not visualized by ERCP because of obliteration or stenosis, the details of the duct were demonstrated by EUS (except in cases of extensive lithiasis).

Pancreatic Duct Branches
Dilated pancreatic duct branches were identified only by ERCP and EUS. This finding occurred in 25 cases (52%) with chronic pancreatitis (Fig. 7-3).

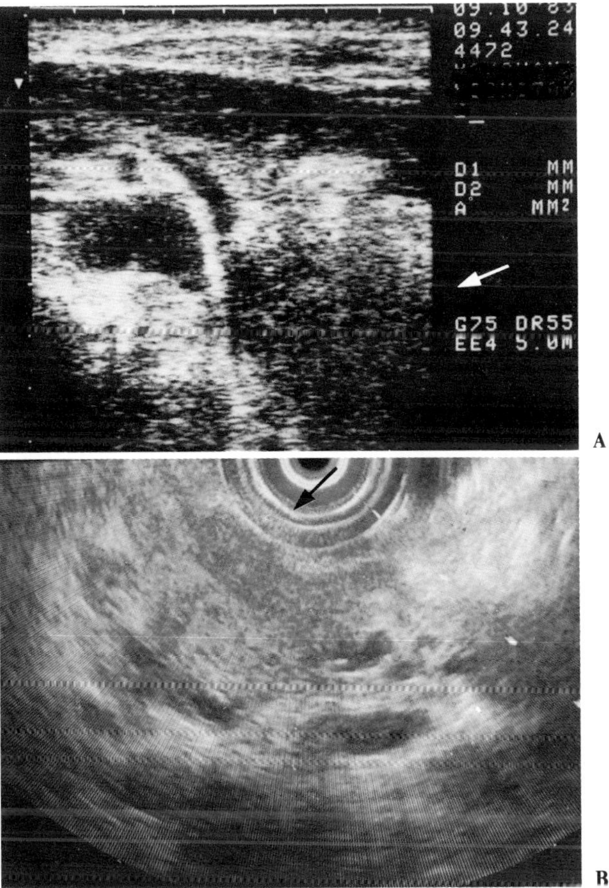

Fig. 7-5. A: Duct cell adenocarcinoma as shown by US. Hypoechoic region is seen in pancreatic tail (arrow). B: Using EUS, a tumor is depicted with lobulated contour and irregular central echoes in the hypoechoic mass (arrow).

Obliteration and Stenosis of Main Pancreatic Duct

Obliteration or stenosis of the MPD was observed by EUS in only five cases, and not clear in four cases. Such findings are important because any abnormality suggesting obliteration or stenosis on EUS leads to further diagnostic examinations (Fig. 7-4).

Solid Space-Occupying Lesions

The main advantage of EUS is its ability to differentiate chronic pancreatitis from pancreatic cancer when conventional imaging methods cannot. Solid space-occupying lesions were detected in seven cases by US, six by EUS, and four by CT. Mass formation was recognized as a localized enlargement and decrease in echo-level by ultrasound. Pseudotumorous pancrea-

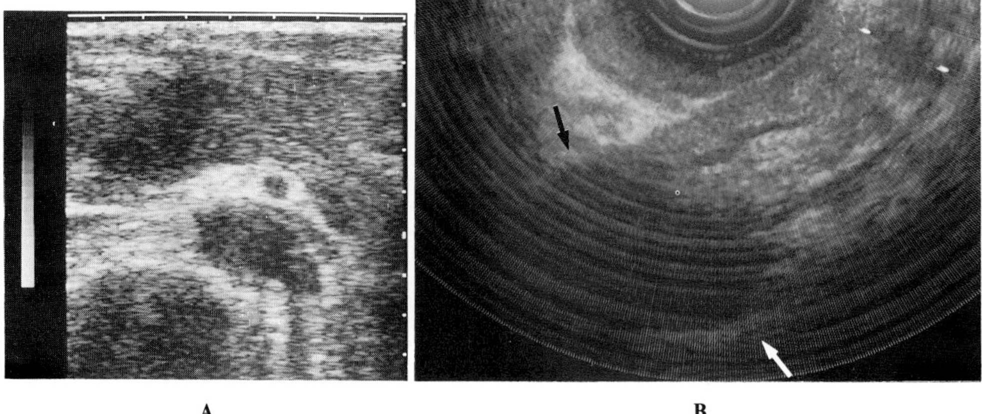

A   B

Fig. 7-6. **A:** Pseudotumorous pancreatitis shown by US. Hypoechoic mass in pancreatic head is seen. **B:** The mass (arrows) has a smooth contour and homogeneous hypoechoic pattern with marked attenuation, as shown by EUS.

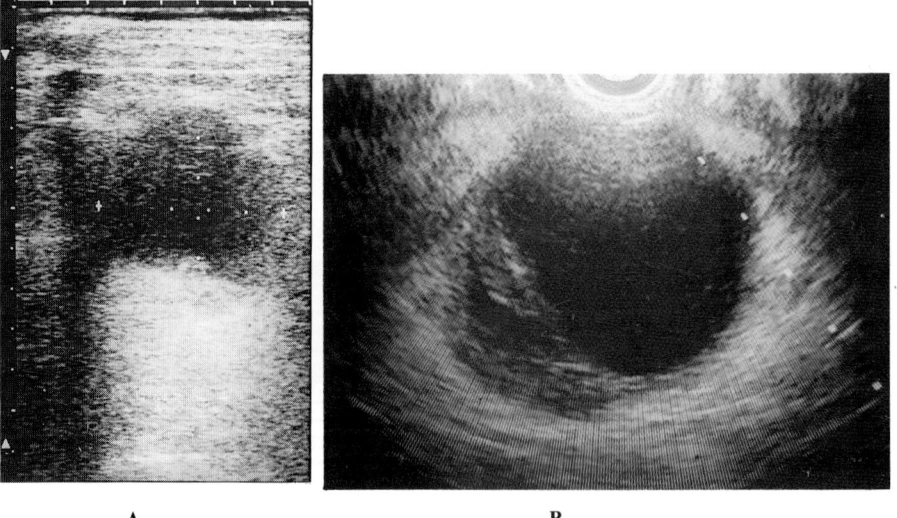

A   B

Fig. 7-7. **A:** Cystadenocarcinoma (tail) as shown by US. Bowel gas obscures the part of the cyst. **B:** With EUS the whole cyst is seen clearly in conjunction with the septum and locally thickened cystwall.

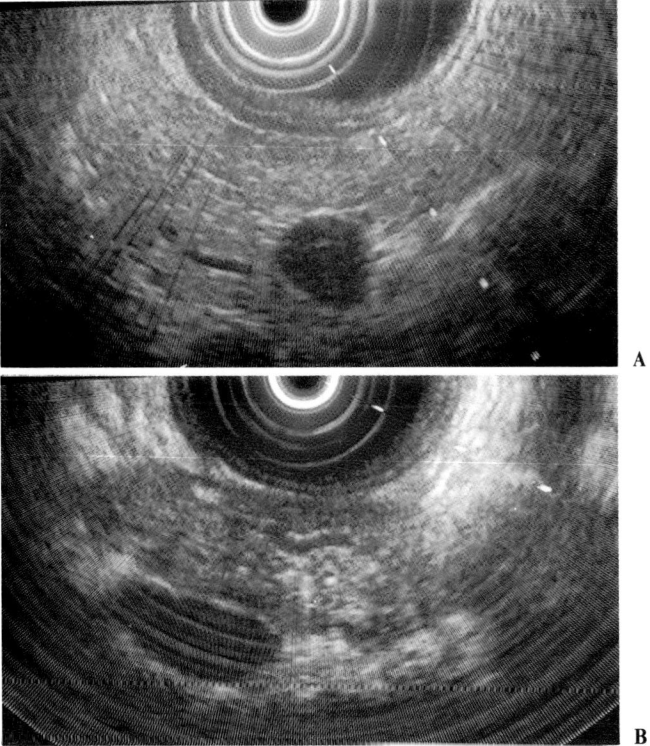

Fig. 7-8. A: Normal pancreas. The parenchyma shows a regularly arranged granular echo-pattern.
B: Chronic pancreatitis. The parenchyma shows a heterogeneous pattern.

titis, which must be differentiated from pancreatic cancer, showed smooth contours and an attenuated homogeneous internal echo-pattern (Fig. 7-5), whereas neoplastic lesions showed irregular contours and a heterogeneous internal echo-pattern (Fig. 7-6). This is especially true when ERCP displays pancreatic duct obstruction or a mass lesion is demonstrated by US or CT. With EUS, one can improve the spatial resolution by using high oscillator frequencies of 7.5 or 10 MHz. This allows clearer imaging of the parenchymal echo-pattern. When the changes are minimal, one may be unable to discern by x-ray CT if a tumor is present or not, but by EUS such minimal changes can be disclosed because of its high-resolution image.

Cyst
Pancreatic cysts that accompanied chronic pancreatitis were observed in eight cases by US (six large, two small), 15 by EUS (seven large, eight small), 12 by CT (seven large, four small), and 13 cases by ERCP (two large, eleven small). ERCP can determine if the cyst communicates with the pancreatic duct. However, one should avoid direct injection of contrast medium into the cyst because of possible complications, such as infection and chemical pancreatitis. When there is no direct communication between the cyst and pancreatic duct it is nearly impossible to delineate the cyst's morphology. The walls and internal structure of cysts can be imaged by either US, EUS, or CT. However, because EUS can visualize all areas of the pancreas with resolution images higher than US or CT, small cysts, cyst wall structure, septa, and cyst fluid are best detected and determined by EUS. The case shown in Fig. 7-7 is cystadenoma compli-

cated with chronic pancreatitis. A partial thickening of the cyst wall and the septum are demonstrated clearly by EUS.

Parenchyma

One of the most important advantages of both ultrasonography and CT is that they visualize the pancreatic parenchyma. Sonographically, the normal pancreatic parenchyma is shown as a fine granular pattern (Fig. 7-8). In this study, a heterogeneous pattern (irregularly arranged) was demonstrated in 32 cases (75%) by EUS. This pattern was noted in 20 of 24 cases (83%) of severe pancreatitis diagnosed by ERCP and in 12 of 22 cases (55%) of mild pancreatitis. EUS using a higher frequency oscillator provides clearer images and is more useful than US in determining pathologic changes in the pancreatic parenchyma with chronic pancreatitis. EUS demonstrates a heterogeneous echo-pattern, which corresponds to parenchymal changes in severe chronic pancreatitis. However, the diagnosis of mild pancreatitis still remains difficult. Further studies will be needed to clarify the relationship and difference between the morphological changes induced by aging and by pathologic alterations in pancreatic function and morphology of chronic pancreatitis.

References

1. Arger PH, Mulhern CB, Bonavita JA, Stauffer DM, Hale J: An analysis of pancreatic sonography in suspected pancreatic disease. J Clin Ultrasound 7: 91–97, 1979.
2. Dimagno EP, Buxton JL, Regan PT, Hattery RR, Wilson DA, Suarez JR, Green PS: Ultrasonic endoscope. Lancet 1: 629–631, 1980.
3. Editorial: Ultrasonography of the pancreas. Lancet 2: 1212–1213, 1977.
4. Lawson TL, Berland LL, Foley WD, Stewart ET, Geenen JE, Hogan WJ: Ultrasonic visualization of the pancreatic duct. Radiology 144: 865–871, 1982.
5. Morita K, Nakazawa S, Naito Y, Kimoto E: Endoscopic ultrasonography of the gallbladder compared with pathological findings. J Jap Gastroenterol 83: 86–95, 1986.
6. Nakazawa S, Sugiyama H, Kimoto E, Naito Y: Specifications of endoscopic ultrasonography. Scand J Gastroenterol 19 (Suppl 94): 1–6, 1984.
7. Strohm WD, Phillip J, Hagenmüller F, Classen M: Ultrasonic tomography by means of ultrasonic fiberscope. Endoscopy 12: 241–244, 1980.
8. Takemoto T, Aibe T, Fuji T, Okita K: Endoscopic Ultrasonography. Clin Gastroenterol 15: 305–319, 1986.
9. Yamanaka T, Sakai H, Yoshida Y, Kawamoto C, Ueno N, Kumagai M, Horiguchi M, Nagasawa S, Tanaka M, Seki H, Ido K, Kimura K: Ultrasonic endoscopy for the abdominal lesions I. Clinical evaluation of an ultrasonic gastroscope with electronic linear scanning system (prototype). Gastroenterol Endosc 24: 598–609, 1982.
10. Yasuda K, Tanaka Y, Fujimoto S, Nakajima M, Kawai K: Use of endoscopic ultrasonography in small pancreatic cancer. Scand J Gastroenterol 19 (Suppl 94) 9–17, 1984.

8

Gallbladder Diseases

Keiichi Morita, Saburo Nakazawa, Eizo Kimoto, Kenji Yamao, and Yoshiki Hahashi

The evolution of ultrasound (US) over the past 20 years has been remarkable. It now plays an important role in diagnosing gallbladder diseases. Despite its advancements, conventional US still has significant limitations because it does not provide images of small gallbladder carcinoma or discriminate from benign diseases, such as cholesterol polyps. Furthermore, it is impossible to determine by US at what stage the disease process is in.

Results of initial endoscopic ultrasonography (EUS) and the continuous improvement of instruments and interpretation have shown that EUS is a more practical technique (1, 4). EUS is now a valuable new dignostic tool in gastroenterology, especially in small pancreatic cancer and small gallbladder cancer (2, 3, 5).

We performed EUS in 18 normal cases in autopsy and 153 clinical cases with gallbladder diseases. From April 1983 to December 1986 we examined by EUS 20 gallbladder cancer

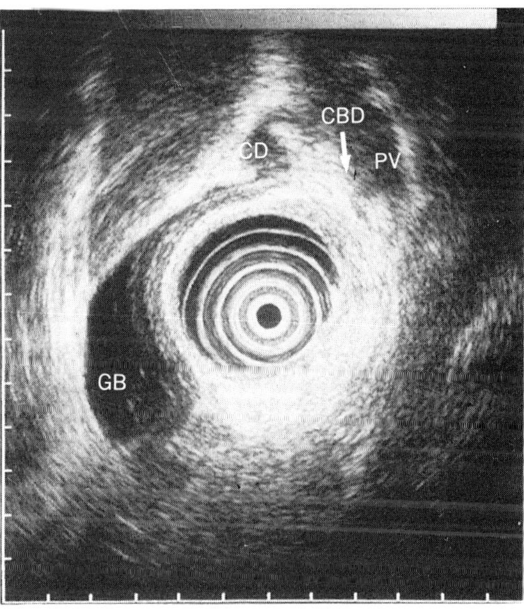

Fig. 8-1. EUS demonstrated clearly the gallbladder (GB), cystic duct (CD), common bile duct (CBD), and portal vein (PV) from bulbus duodeni.

Table 8-1. Visualization rate of gallbladder by US and EUS in 90 clinical cases.

	Neck	Body	Fundus
US	84/90 (93.3%)	90/90 (100%)	57/90 (63.3%)
EUS	88/90 (97.8%)	88/90 (97.8%)	82/90 (91.1%)

cases, 57 cholesterol polyp cases, 20 adenomyomatosis cases, 49 cholecystolithiasis cases, and seven cholecystitis cases.

In all patients, we carried out US with a Toshiba SAL-30A, 3.5 MHz or a Toshiba SSA-90A, 3.75 MHz ultrasound tomograph, followed by EUS. The instruments used in this study were the third and fourth type of EUS with a 7.5 MHz and/or 10 MHz rotating transducer (Olympus GF-UM1, GF-UM2). Premedication for EUS is the same as that for upper gastrointestinal tract endoscopy (lidocaine pharyngeal anesthesia and intramuscular injection of butropium bromide). After premedication, the patients were studied in the left lateral position. For better visualization, 15 to 20 ml of deaerated water was instilled into the balloon of the EUS tip. In the bulbus duodeni, the gallbladder usually was demonstrated (Fig. 8-1). Comparing the detecting capability of the gallbladder parts in 90 clinical cases, EUS was superior to US in detecting all parts of the gallbladder (Table 8-1).

In this chapter we compared echograms and the histological findings of gallblader diseases obtained by US and EUS.

GALLBLADDER WALL

NORMAL GALLBLADDER WALL

EUS demonstrated the gallbladder wall as three layers in clinical examinations as well as the normal autopsy specimen, which has no gallbladder lesions in the water bath (Fig. 8-2). The comparison between findings by EUS and histology revealed the tissue components matched with these ultrasonographical layers. The first and most inner layer with a slightly hypoechoic level corresponded with the mucosal layer; the second middle thin layer and the hypoechoic layer implicated the muscular layer; the third outer hyperechoic layer represented the serosal and subserosal layers.

WALL OF ADENOMYOMATOSIS

The gallbladder wall of adenomyomatosis was demonstrated as type III (Table 8-2). The gallbladder wall in the case of adenomyomatosis came into sight as two layers comprising a low echoic and thick layer and another high echoic layer, and small cystic echoes in the gallbladder wall. On the histological findings, muscle and growing perimuscular fibrosis matched the low echoic and thick layer.

WALL OF CHOLECYSTITIS AND GALLBLADDER STONE

The gallbladder wall of cholecystitis and gallbladder stone was thick and usually was visualized

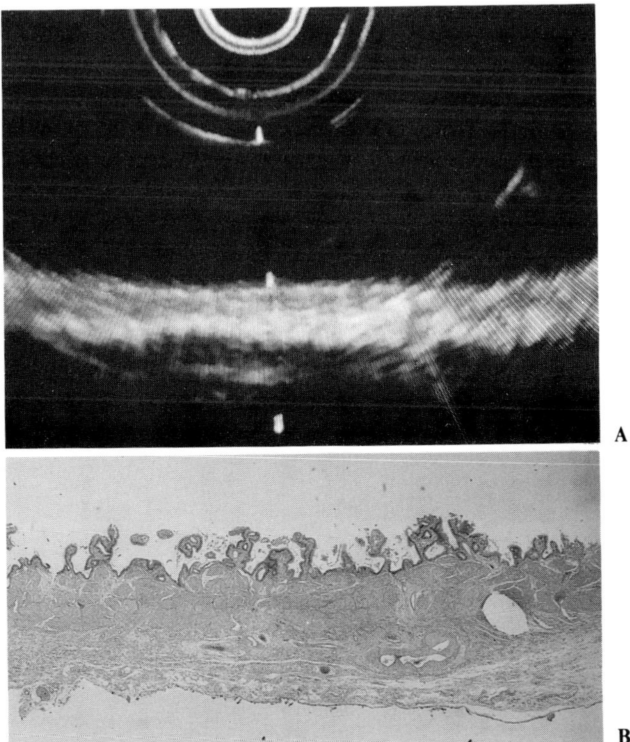

Fig. 8-2. By EUS the gallbladder wall was demonstrated as three layers in the autopsy specimen in the water bath. Comparison between EUS (**A**) and histology (**B**) revealed which tissue components corresponded to these ultrasonic layers. The first slightly hyperechoic layer represented the mucosal layer, the second thin hypoechoic layer implicated the muscular layer, and the third hyperechoic layer matched the serosal and subserosal layers.

Table 8-2. Comparison between endoscopic ultrasonograms and pathological findings in 48 resected cases.

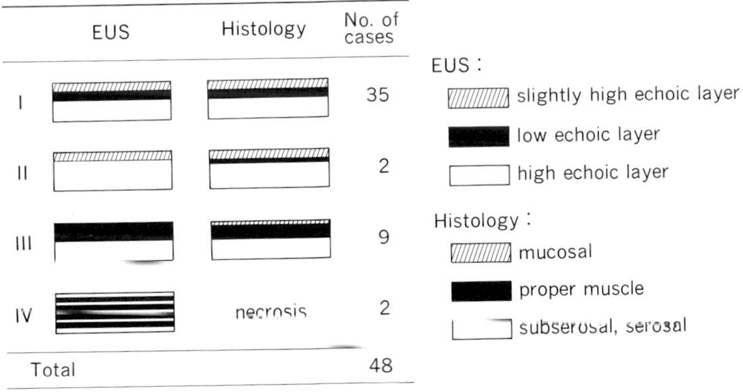

by EUS as three or more layers (Table 8-2). In severe cholecystitis the gallbladder wall was thick and separated into multiple layers (type IV; Table 8-2). US and EUS demonstrated stones in the gallbladder, but the shadow of the stone was more clearly demonstrated by EUS than by US (see Fig. 8-7).

BENIGN DISEASE

CHOLESTEROL POLYP

Comparing US and EUS echograms of resected gallbladder cholesterol polyps (Table 8-3), most of the small cholesterol polyps were demonstrated by US as homogeneous hyperechoic masses. Five of the eight large cholesterol polyps were visualized as the multiple granular structure comprising hyperechoic spots, but the other polyps were not.

EUS provided a clear view of the cholesterol polyps in the gallbladder as the multiple granular structure comprising hyperechoic spots. All the gallbladder walls in the cholesterol polyps were demonstrated as three layers by EUS as well as normal gallbladder wall of autopsy specimen (Figs. 8-2 and 8-3). On the histological findings, the group of foamy cells showed granular structures, and its histological findings matched that of the EUS findings (Fig. 8-3).

Because of better resolusion with EUS, all the cholesterol polyps in the gallbladder were demonstrated as a multiple granular structure comprising hyperechoic spots (hyperechoic multigranular structure), whereas US did not allow such a demonstration (2).

Table 8-3. Comparison of echograms of the gallbladder cholesterol polyps between US and EUS.

Size of polyp	US	EUS	No. of cases
10 mm >	2		
	2	8	8
	4		
10 mm ≤	3		
15 mm ≥	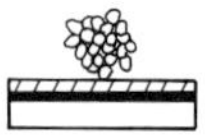 3	6	6
15 mm <	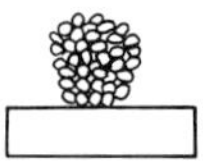 2 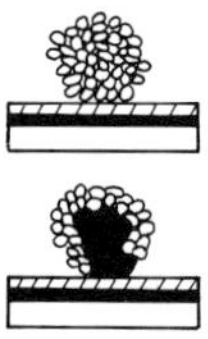	1	2
		1	
Total			16

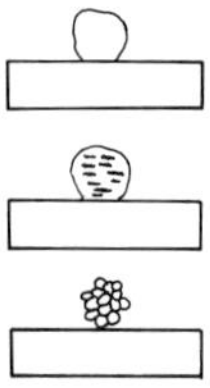

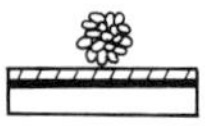

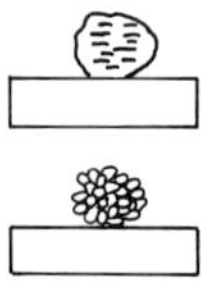

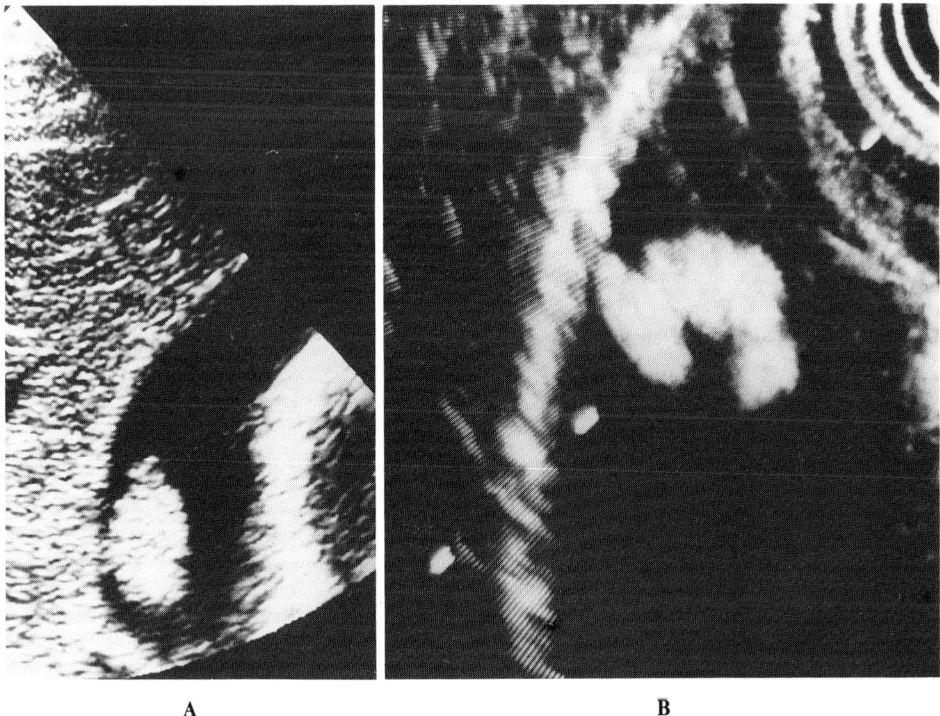

A   B

Fig. 8-3. US (**A**) and EUS (**B**) of the cholesterol polyp in the gallbladder. EUS clearly showed the cholesterol polyps in the gallbladder as the multiple granular structure comprising hyperechoic spots, whereas US did not.

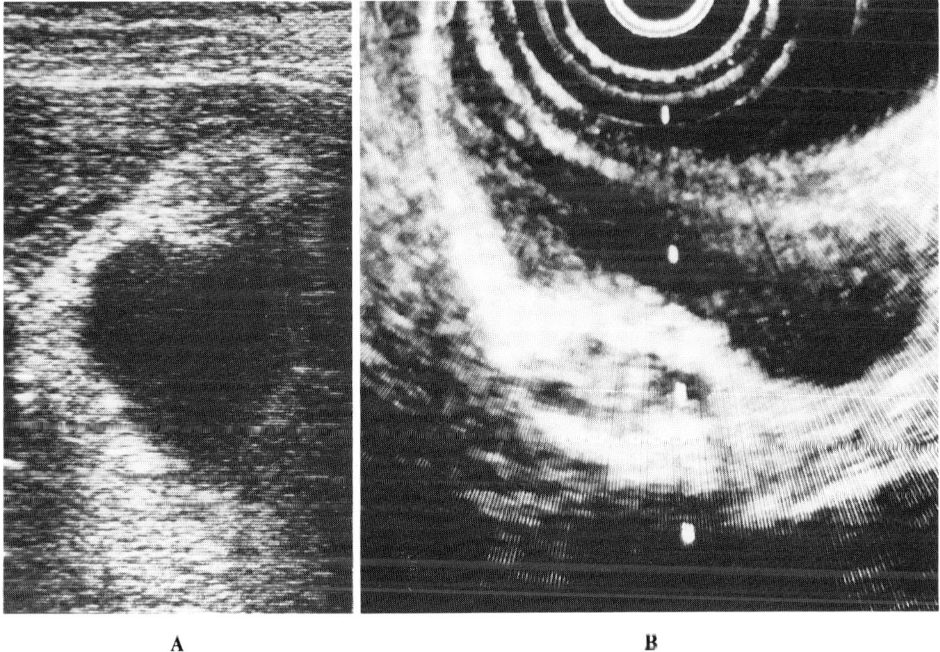

A   B

Fig. 8-4. US (**A**) and EUS (**B**) of the fundal type of gallbladder adenomyomatosis. EUS clearly demonstrated the polypoid lesions as the gallbladder wall thickness with cystic echoes, which corresponded histologically with RA-sinus.

Table 8-4. Comparison of echograms of the gallbladder polypoid lesions between US and EUS.

	Size of polyp	US		EUS		No. of cases
Gallbladder adenomyomatosis 2	10 mm ≦ 15 mm ≧		2		2	2
Gallbladder cancer 10	10 mm >		1		1	1
	10 mm ≦		2		m 1 pm 1	3
	15 mm ≧		1		m 1	
	15 mm <		6		pm 2 ss 1 s 3	6
Total						12

m: mucosal; pm: proper muscle; ss: subserosal; s: serosal.

Table 8-5. Endoscopic ultrasonographical findings of the gallbladder carcinoma.

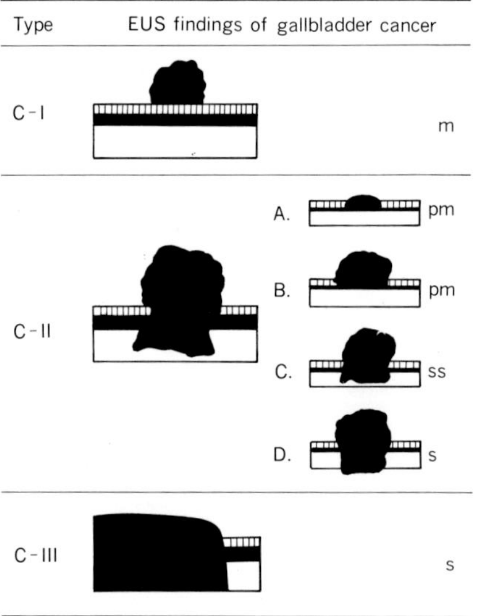

Type C-I: A fungating mass on the gallbladder wall without the destruction of the gallbladder wall. Type C-II: A protuberant mass on the gallbladder wall and irregular hypoechoic mass in the gallbladder wall caused by infiltration of carcinoma. Type C-III: Homogeneous hypoechoic thickening of the gallbladder wall caused by infiltration of carcinoma.

m: mucosal; pm: proper muscle; ss: subserosal; s: serosal.

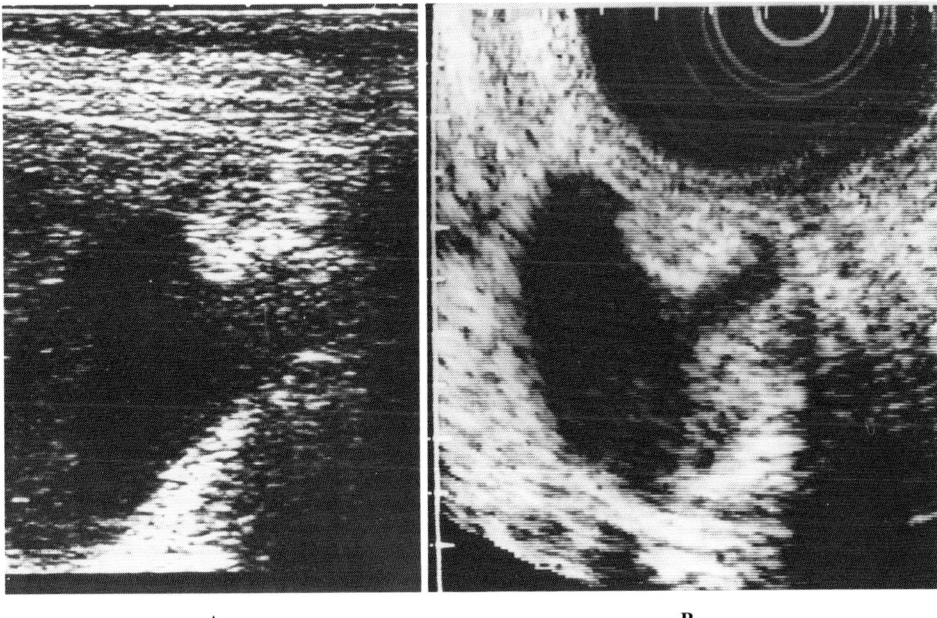

Fig. 8-5. US (**A**) and EUS (**B**) of the polypoid type of early gallbladder cancer. By EUS the gallbladder wall was visualized to three layers and the gallbladder wall in which the gallbladder cancer appeared was visualized to three layers. Therefore, the depth of the cancer's infiltration of the gallbladder wall was diagnosed to emanate from the mucus layer.

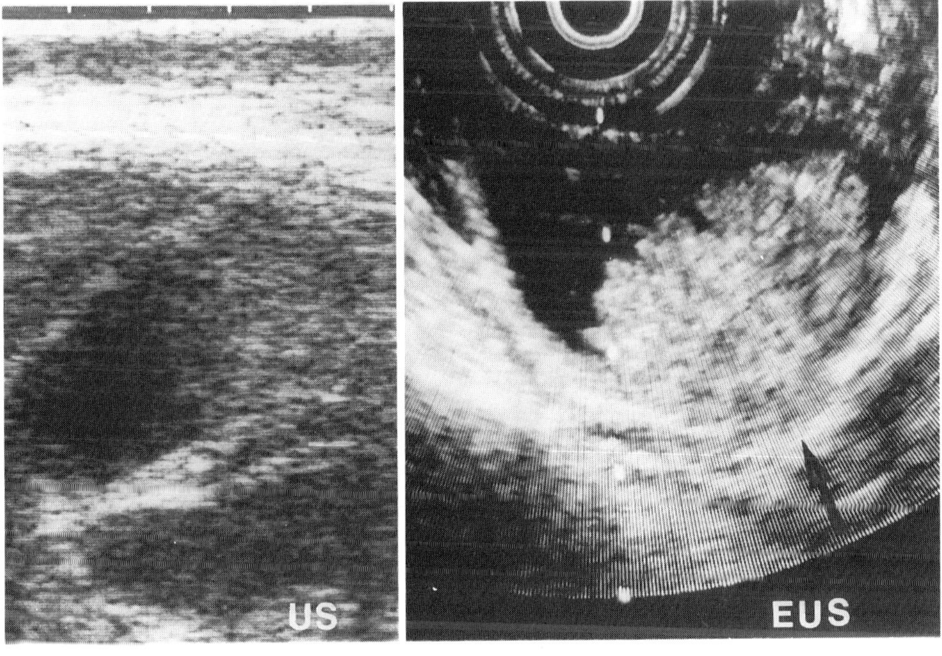

Fig. 8-6. US (**A**) and EUS (**B**) of the polypoid type of advanced gallbladder cancer. Only by EUS was the infiltration to the gallbladder wall clearly demonstrated as the destruction of three layers of the gallbladder wall (arrow). The shape of the tumor was visualized as a papillary irregular hypoechoic mass by EUS. This irregular growth was not detected by US.

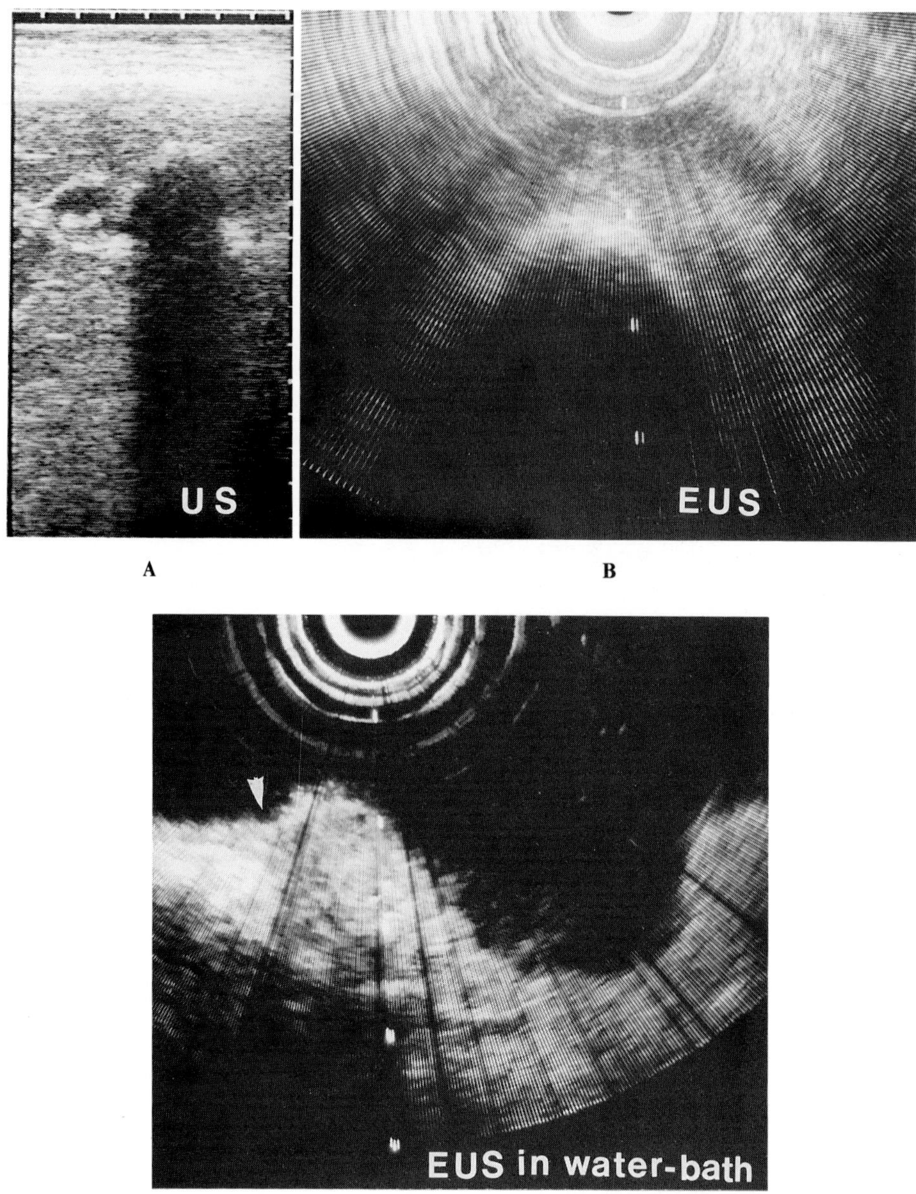

Fig. 8-7. The EUS sonogram (**B**) demonstrated homogeneous hypoechoic thickening of the gallbladder wall, which was not shown clearly by US (**A**). Gallstones and acoustic shadowing were apparent in EUS. EUS in the water bath (**C**) demonstrated tumor infiltration in the wall of the resected gallbladder specimen.

ADENOMYOMATOSIS

We compared US and EUS echograms of resected gallbladder polypoid lesions (Table 8-4). EUS made it possible to identify the protruding lesions of the polypoid type of gallbladder adenomyomatosis as polypoid lesions with small cystic echoes in the gallbladder wall. US did not identify them (Fig. 8-4).   On the histological findings, the lesions of adenomyomatosis have many dilated Rokitanski-Ashoff sinuses (RA-sinuses); the findings of the dilated RA-sinus corresponded with the EUS findings of the small cystic echoes in the gallbladder wall (2).

GALLBLADDER CANCER

EUS allowed a clear view of the polypoid type of gallbladder carcinoma as a papillary, irregular, and low echoic mass (Tables 8-4 and 8-5).   Such an irregular growth was not detected by US. The tumor infiltration into the gallbladder wall was clearly demonstrated by EUS as destruction of three layers of the gallbladder wall, wereas it was not discerned by US (Figs. 8-5 and 8-6).

EUS provided useful information regarding the differential diagnosis of cholecystitis and the wall-thickened type of gallbladder cancer (Table 8-5).   The gallbladder wall, free from inflammation or with moderate inflammation, was separated into three layers by EUS (type I; Table 8-2), and the gallbladder wall of severe cholecystitis was separated into many layers (type IV; Table 8-2).   However, the gallbladder wall of the gallbladder cancer was visualized as a homogeneous low echoic layer (type C-III; Table 8-5, Fig. 8-7).

The most important diagnostic aspects of EUS investigation of gallbladder disease are differential diagnosis of gallbladder lesions as well as determination of the depth of tumor infiltration in the gallbladder wall.   In gallbladder carcinoma, infiltration to the gallbladder wall was clearly demonstrated by EUS as the destruction of three layers of the gallbladder wall (Table 8-5).

References

1.   Dimagno EP, Buxton JI, Regan PT, Hattery RR, Wilson DA, Suarez JR, Green PS: Ultrasonic endoscope.   Lancet 1: 629–631, 1980.
2.   Morita K, Nakazawa S, Naito Y, Kimoto E, Inui K, Ohnuma T: Endoscopic ultrasonography in the diagnosis of gallbladder disease.   In Gill RW, Dadd MJ (eds): Proceedings of the Fourth Meeting of the World Federation for Ultrasound in Medicine and Biology (WFUMB) and the First World Congress of Sonographers, Sydney, 1985, p 145.
3.   Nakazawa S, Sugiyama H, Kimoto E, Naito Y: Specification of endoscopic ultrasonography in small pancreatic cancer.   Scand J Gastroenterol 19 (102): 1–6, 1984.
4.   Strohm WD, Phillip J. Hagenmüller F, Classen M: Ultrasonic tomography by means of an ultrasonic fiberscope.   Endoscopy 12: 241–244, 1980.
5.   Yasuda K, Tanaka Y, Fujimoto S, Nakajima M, Kawai K: Use of endoscopic ultrasonography in small pancreatic cancer.   Scand J Gastroenterol 19 (102): 9–17, 1984.

9
Diseases of the Biliary Tract and the Papilla of Vater

Kenjiro Yasuda, Masatsugu Nakajima, and Keiichi Kawai

The use of body-imaging diagnostics for diagnosing biliary tract and papilla of Vater diseases has become common since the development of endoscopic retrograde cholangiopancreatography (ERCP) (4). ERCP is an endoscopic technique that enables us to diagnose the diseases of the pancreatobiliary tract on x-ray film. New techniques using ERCP, such as endoscopic sphincterotomy (EST) (6), endoscopic retrograde biliary drainage (ERBD) (9), and peroral cholangiopancreatoscopy (PCPS) (8) are now in clinical use. However, ERCP and other techniques using ERCP sometimes are invasive, and they cannot be performed by all physicians.

Conventional ultrasonography (US) has become widespread in the past several years as a noninvasive screening test. This technique was first thought to be the ultimate diagnostic method for diseases of the hepatopancreatobiliary tract, but it was discovered to have limitations in diagnosing these lesions because of the echoic reduction induced by subcutaneous

Table 9-1. Biliary tract diseases examined by endoscopic ultrasonography.

Common bile duct			33
Cancer	10		
≤ 20 mm		5	
$20 < \; \leqq 30$ mm		4	
$30 <$		1	
Adenoma	1		
≤ 20 mm		1	
Dilatation	3		
Stone	19		
Papilla of Vater			17
Cancer	9		
≤ 20 mm		4	
$20 < \; \leqq 30$ mm		3	
30 mm $<$		2	
Papillary stenosis	8		
Gallbladder			70
Cancer	8		
$20 < \; \leqq 30$ mm		1	
30 mm $<$		7	
Adenoma	3		
≤ 20 mm		3	
Cholesterol polyp	36		
Adenomyomatosis	7		
Stone with cholecystitis	14		
Others	2		
Total			120 cases

fatty tissue, bones, intestinal gas, and the anatomically deeper position of the pancreas and biliary tract. Endoscopic ultrasonography (EUS) was developed to overcome these problems, and for the early diagnosis of pancreatobiliary cancer by intra digestive canal ultrasonographic scanning (1, 3, 5, 7, 11, 12, 14, 16). EUS uses a higher frequency, thus allowing precise ultrasonographic imaging because the position of the transducer is adjacent to the target organs.

In this chapter we will describe EUS diagnosis of the biliary tract and the papilla of Vater. Table 9-1 shows the cases of biliary tract diseases examined by EUS.

BILIARY TRACT, MAINLY IN THE BILE DUCT

NORNAL ENDOSCOPIC ULTRASONOGRAPHIC IMAGE OF THE BILIARY TRACT

For EUS scanning of the biliary tract, it is recommended that the echo-endoscope be inserted up to the duodenum and an ultrasonographic scan be performed through the water-filled balloon covering the tip of the scope that comes into contact with the duodenal wall. By careful EUS scanning through the duodenal wall, the EUS image of the whole bile duct can be observed with the right lobe of the liver, the portal vein (PV) and the pancreas head as reference organs. Fig. 9-1 shows the EUS image of the entire bile duct as observed from the second portion of the duodenum using the balloon-contact method. The image of the gallbladder is obtainable through the wall of the duodenal bulbus or the gastric prepyrolus. The images of the portal vein and the splenic vein, important vessels in discussing the invasion of cancer of the biliary tract, also are detectable through the duodenal or gastric walls. Fig. 9-2 shows the standard scanning position and EUS images schematically.

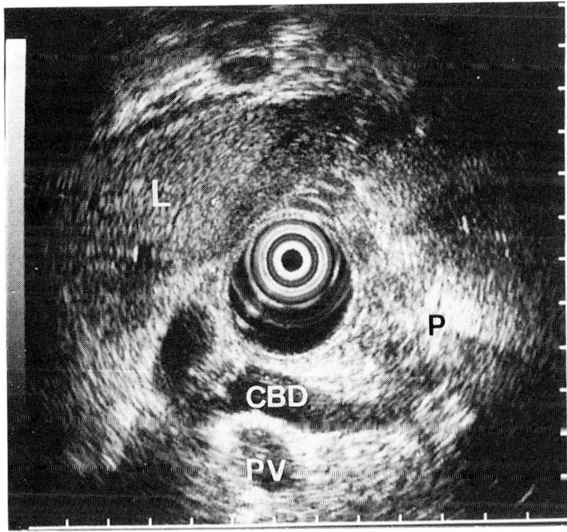

Fig. 9-1. An image of the biliary tract through the duodenal wall using EUS. CBD: common bile duct; L: liver; P: pancreas; PV: portal vein.

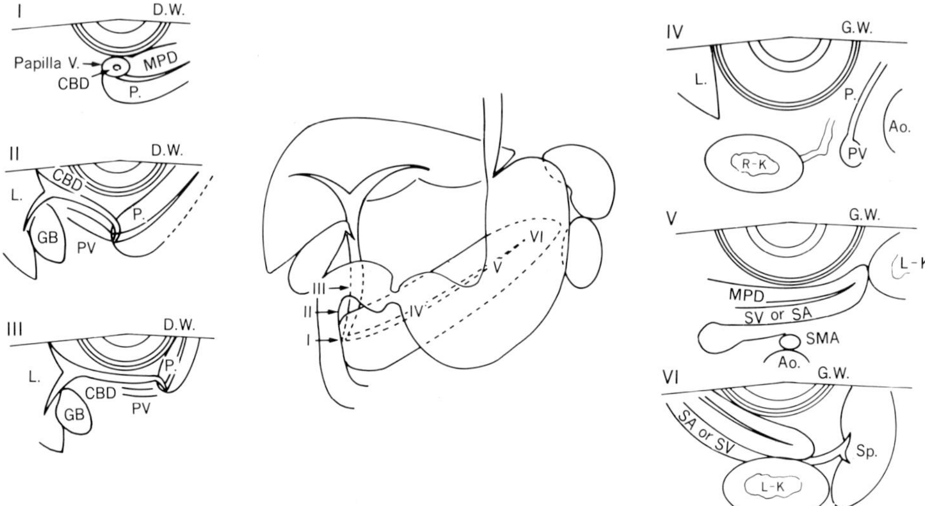

Fig. 9-2. The standard scanning images and preferable approach of EUS for the observation of the biliary tract and pancreas. L.: liver; CBD: common bile duct; GB: gall bladder; P.: pancreas; R-K: right kidney; L-K: left kidney; Sp.: spleen; Ao: Aorta; SMA: superior mesenteric artery; PV: portal vein; SV(A): splenic vein (artery); D.W.: duodenal wall; G.W.: gastric wall.

BILIARY TRACT DISEASES

Benign Diseases

Gallstones are a common product of the biliary tract, and easily detected by US. However, the detection of choledochal stones by US is not always successful because of the disturbance caused by the presence of the intestine and deeper position of the bile dut. EUS, which can observe the bile duct from a close position, provides a clear echogram especially at the end of the bile duct. Fig. 9-3 shows an EUS image of a gallstone. For choledochal stones, ERCP is the preferred approach for performing EST and for the removal of the stones. However, EUS is useful for detecting a stone at the end of the bile duct (Fig. 9-4), as well as for the differential diagnosis of gallbladder polyps, cholesterol polyps, and adenoma. Fig. 9-5 shows a US and EUS image of adenoma in the gallbladder.

Malignant Lesions in the Biliary Tract

US can easily image advanced cancers in the biliary tract but it and computed tomography (CT) have difficulty in detecting cancers in their early stages. ERCP is a valuable technique in the detection of lesions of the bile duct delineating the intracanal space. EUS can provide the ultrasonographic images of the tumor clearly even if the diameter of the tumor is smaller than 10 mm.

Fig. 9-6 shows a case of middle bile duct cancer delineating the hypoechoic mass together with liver, portal vein, terminal bile duct, and pancreas head. This EUS image can provide information regarding the size of the tumor and its invasion into the blood vessels. In the case of cancer at the terminal end of the bile duct, the tumor mass is depicted more clearly by EUS than by US or CT (Fig. 9-7). EUS can detect bile duct cancer more often than other body-imaging diagnostics (such as US, CT, and angiography). This is especially true in the case of tumors smaller than 30 mm in diameter (Table 9-2). ERCP provides as high a detection rate

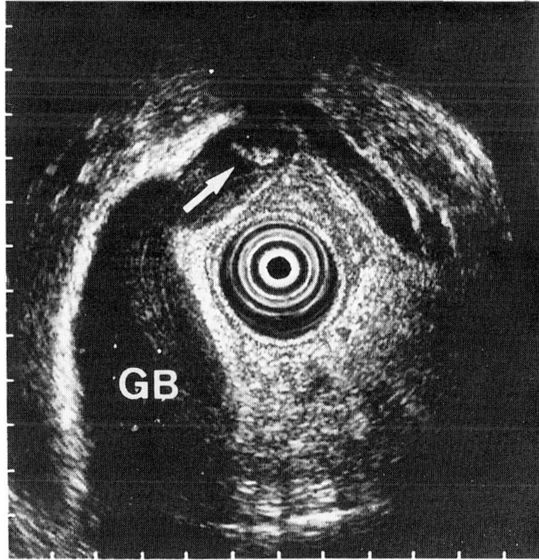

Fig. 9-3. An EUS image of a gallstone (arrow) at the neck of the gallbladder (GB).

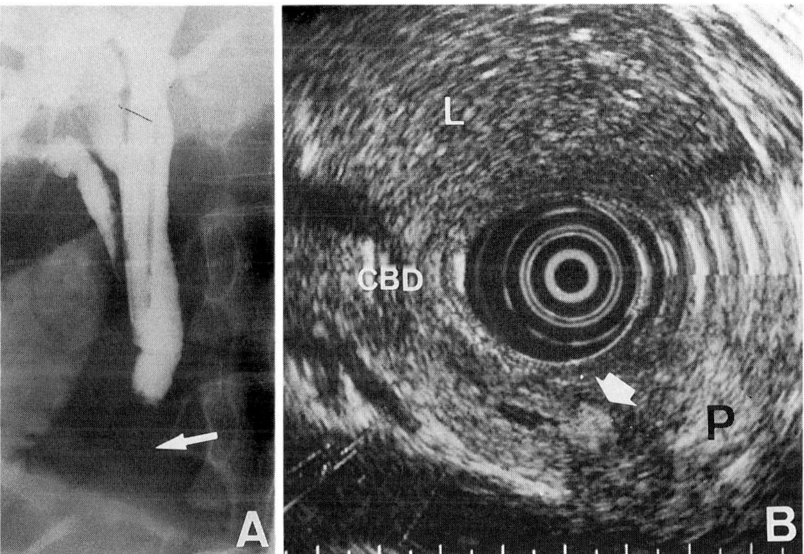

Fig. 9-4. A choledochal stone. **A.** Percutaneous transhepatic cholangiography (PTC) shows the irregular obstruction at the terminal end of the common bile duct (CBD) (arrow). It was difficult to diagnose whether it was a stone or a cancer. **B.** Using EUS, a hypoechoic echogram of the stone is detected at the intrapancreatic bile duct (arrow). L: liver; P: pancreas.

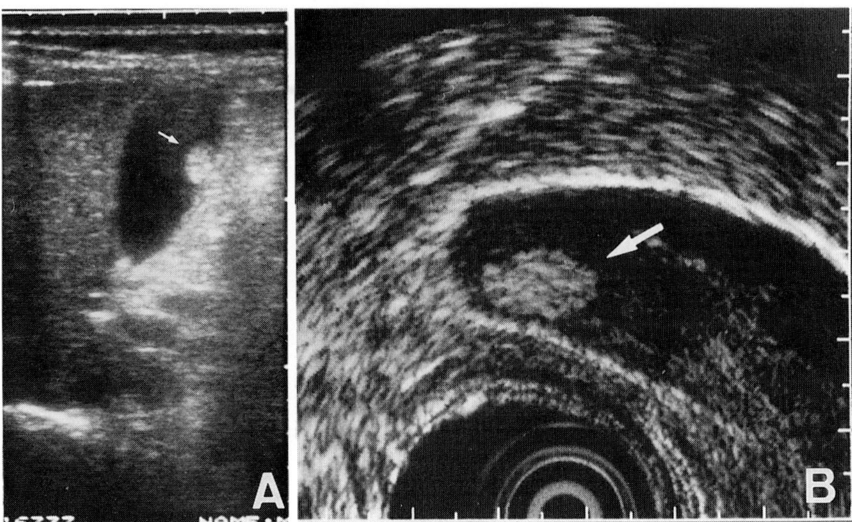

Fig. 9-5. An EUS image of a polyp of the gallbladder compared with an image of US. **A.** The image of the gallbladder adenoma (arrow) using US. **B.** The image of the gallbladder adenoma (arrow) using EUS.

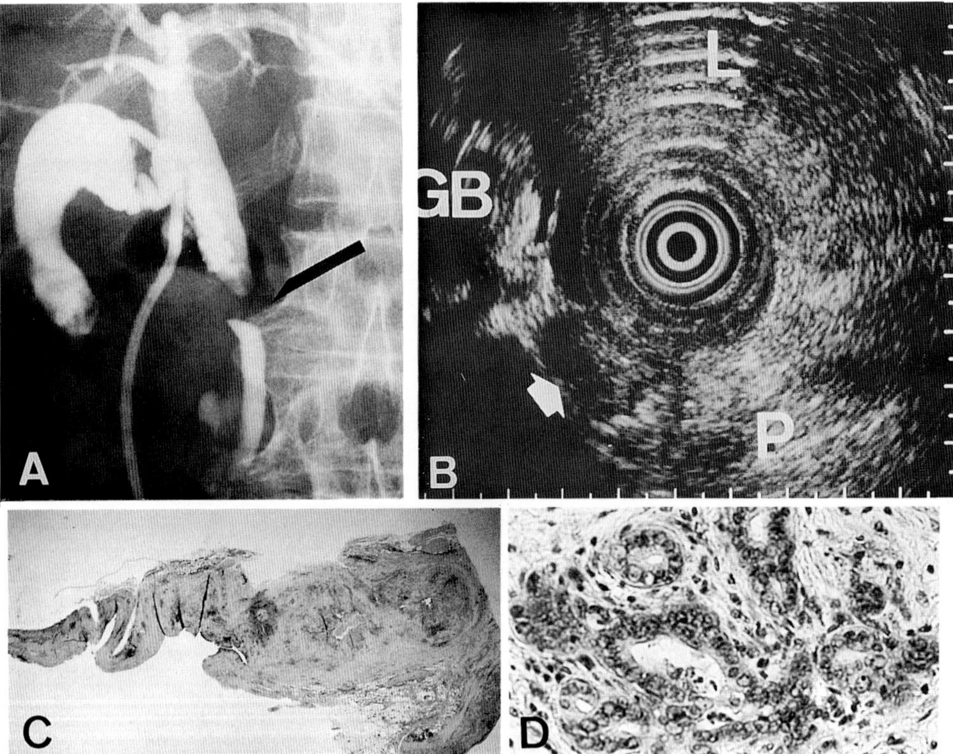

Fig. 9-6. Middle bile duct cancer. **A.** PTC finding shows a filling defect at the middle bile duct involving the cystic duct (arrow). **B.** EUS image through the duodenal wall shows the hypoechoic tumor (22 × 15 mm in diameter) (arrow) at the middle bile duct with a dilated higher bile duct and a normal lower bile duct. GB: gallbladder; P: pancreas. **C, D.** Histological findings show an adenocarcinoma of the bile duct.

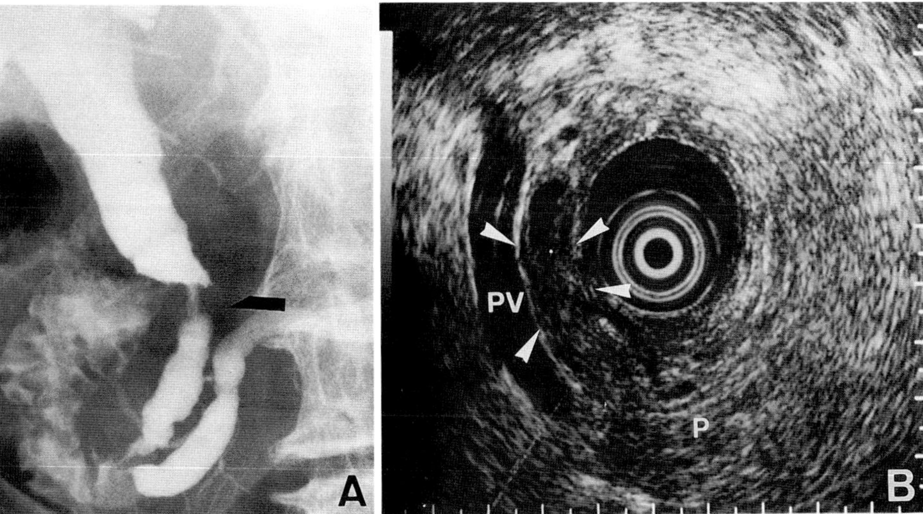

Fig. 9-7.   Bile duct cancer at the terminal end of the common bile duct. **A**. Endoscopic retrograde cholangiography shows a stenosis at the terminal end of the common bile duct (arrow). **B**. EUS image through the duodenal wall shows the hypoechoic tumor mass (14 × 8 mm in diameter) (arrow). Histologically, it was revealed to be an adenocarcinoma of the bile duct. P: pancreas; PV: portal vein.

Table 9-2.   The capability of various body-imaging diagnostics to detect the tumor of the bile duct smaller than 30 mm in diameter.

	EUS	US	ERCP	CT	Angiography
Bile duct	10/10	5/10	10/10	4/10	5/10

as EUS, but can detect only the filling defect or stenotic change of the bile duct rather than the tumor mass itself or neighboring organs. Therefore, the use of the combined images of EUS and ERCP is the preferred method for detecting small lesions in the biliary tract.

PAPILLA OF VATER

NORMAL ENDOSCOPIC ULTRASONOGRAPHIC IMAGE OF THE PAPILLA OF VATER

The EUS image of papilla of Vater is obtained from the second portion of the duodenal wall by contacting the water-filled balloon with the papilla of Vater. Fig. 9-8 shows the EUS image of papilla of Vater with the terminal bile duct and pancreatic duct. An ultrasonogram of a normal papilla of Vater cannot be obtained by other body-imaging diagnostics. Furthermore, a direct view of the papilla is obtained by EUS.

DISEASES OF THE PAPILLA OF VATER

Benign Lesions
Benign lesions of the papilla of Vater, except for papillitis (papillary stenosis), are rare. The EUS image of papillitis shows no abnormalities except for swelling.

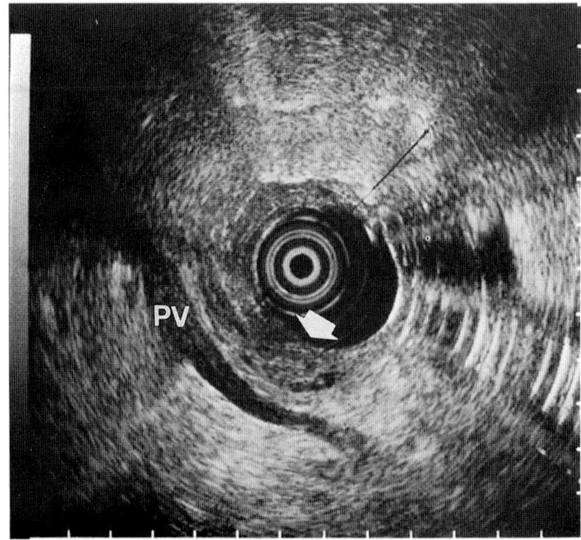

Fig. 9-8. An EUS image of the normal papilla of Vater (arrow) obtained by the EUS scanning on the papilla of Vater. PV: portal vein.

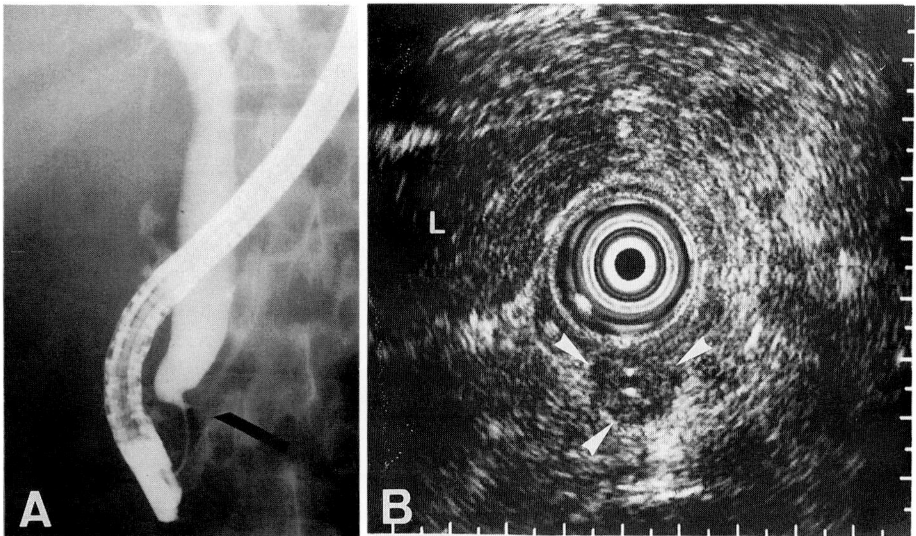

Fig. 9-9. Cancer of the papilla of Vater. **A.** Endoscopic retrograde cholangiography shows an irregular stenosis at the pancreatobiliary junction (arrow). **B.** EUS image shows a hypoechoic tumoral swelling of the papilla of Vater (arrow heads). L: liver.

Malignant lesions

The EUS image of cancer of the papilla shows a characteristic change with or without expansion into the bile duct or pancreas head. Fig. 9-9 shows the ERCP and EUS findings of small papilla cancer to be a solid mass. Fig. 9-10 shows a case of papilla cancer infiltrating the bile duct and pancreas with a diffuse hypoechoic lesion. Diagnosis of the growth of papilla cancer

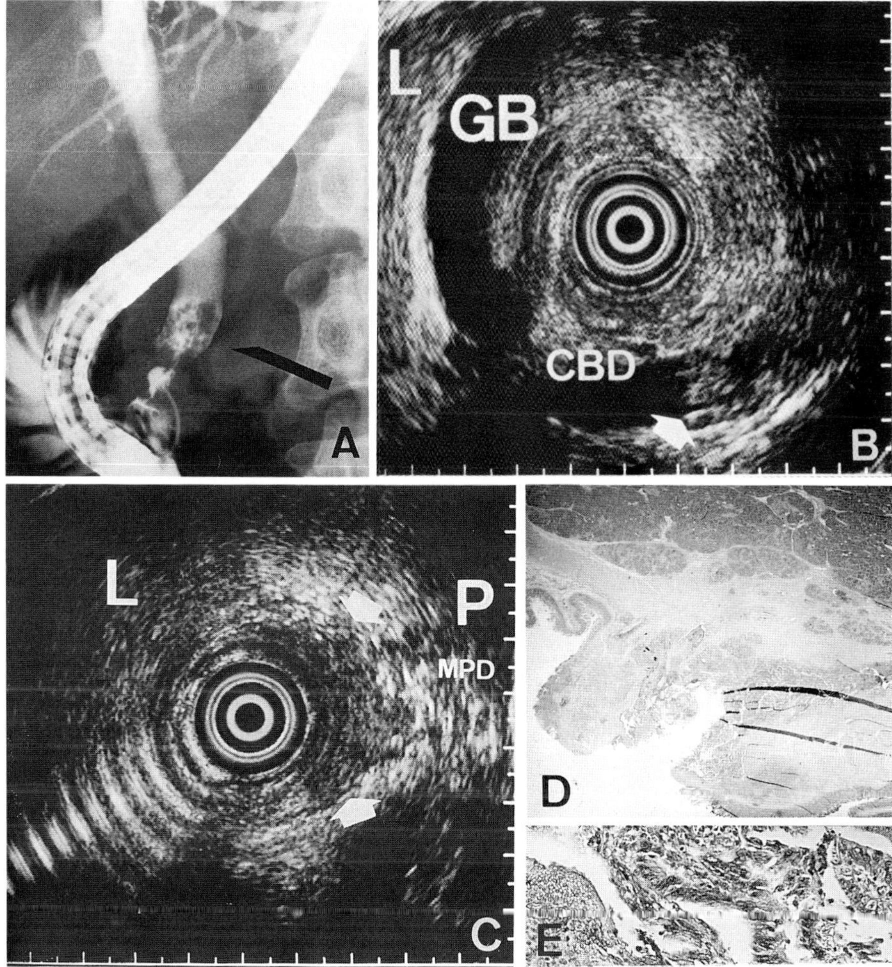

Fig. 9-10. Cancer of the papilla of Vater. **A.** Endoscopic retrograde cholangiography shows the stenosis and irregular filling defect at the terminal end of the common bile duct (arrow). **B.** EUS image through the duodenal wall shows the tumor echogram in the common bile duct (CBD) (arrow). GB: gallbladder. **C.** EUS image on the papilla of Vater shows an irregular hypoechoic tumor (arrow). L: liver; MPD: main pancreatic duct; P: pancreas. **D, E.** Histological findings show an adenocarcinoma of the papilla of Vater.

Table 9-3. The capability of various body-imaging diagnostics to detect the cancer of papilla of Vater smaller than 30 mm in diameter

	EUS	US	ERCP	CT	Angiography
Papilla of Vater	7/7	1/7	7/7	2/6	1/6

is difficult by conventional diagnostics. Table 9-3 shows the capability of various imaging diagnostics to detect cancer of the papilla of Vater. These results show that EUS is the most useful method in the detection of the tumor mass as well as in the diagnosis of the expansion into the bile duct and pancreas.

SUMMARY

The development of ERCP and US examinations has made diseases of the biliary tract and the papilla of Vater easier to diagnose. However, it is still difficult to detect the tumor and its invasion accurately. By using EUS, lesions of the biliary tract and papilla of Vater are delineated with an ultrasonographic image from a closer position. These EUS images of biliary tract diseases have revolutionized the field by making available for the first time high-frequency ultrasonographic images and the ultrasonographic visualization of the papilla of Vater (2, 10, 13, 15). In addition, with EUS, the expansion of the lesion and its resectability can be discussed accurately, especially in the case of small lesions. Table 9-4 shows the role of EUS in the diagnosis of biliary tract diseases. The improvement of the echo-endoscope with a channel to make an ERCP examination is awaited.

Table 9-4. The role of EUS in the diagnosis of biliary tract diseases.

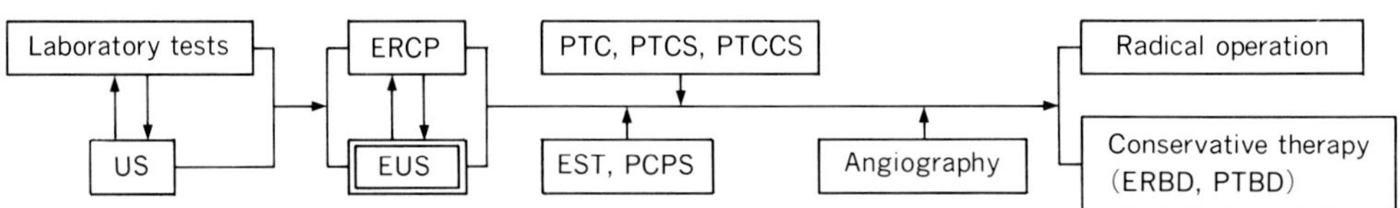

PTCS: Percutaneous transhepatic cholangioscopy; PTCCS: Percutaneous transhepatic cholecystoscopy; PCPS: Peroral cholangiopancreatoscopy.

References

1. Classen M, Strohm WD, Kurtz W: Pancreatic pseudocysts and tumors in endosonography. Scand J Gastroenterol 19 (Suppl 94): 77–84, 1984.
2. Dancygier H, Classen M: Endosonographic diagnosis of benign pancreatic and biliary lesions. Scan J Gastroenterol 21 (Suppl 123): 119–122, 1986.
3. Fukuda M, Nakano Y, Saito K, Hirata K, Terada S, Urushizaki I: Endoscopic ultrasonography in the diagnosis of pancreatic carcinoma: The use of a liquid-filled stomach method. Scand J Gastroenterol 19 (Suppl 94): 65–76, 1984.
4. Fukumoto K, Nakajima M, Murakami K, Kawai K: Diagnosis of pancreatic cancer by endoscopic pancreatocholangiography. Am J Gastroenterol 62: 210–213, 1974.
5. Heyder N, Lutz H, Lux G, Demling L: Initial results of transgastric endoscopic ultrasonography in comparison with external ultrasound. Scand J Gastroenterol 19 (Suppl 94) 85–90, 1984.
6. Kawai K, Nakajima M, Kimoto K: Endoscopic sphincterotomy of the ampulla of Vater. Gastrointest Endosc 20: 148–151, 1974.
7. Lux G, Heyder N: Endoscopic ultrasonography of the pancreas: Technical aspects. Scand J Gastroenterol 21 (Suppl 123): 112–118, 1986.
8. Nakajima M, Akasaka Y, Fukumoto K, Mitsuyoshi Y, Kawai K: Peroral cholangiopancreatoscopy (PCPS) under duodenoscopic guidance. Am J Gastroenterol 66: 241–247, 1976.
9. Soehendra N, Reynders-Frendrix V: Palliative bile duct drainage: A new endoscopic method of introducing a transpapillary drainage. Endoscopy 12: 8–11, 1980.
10. Strohm WD, Kurtz W, Classen M: Detection of biliary stones by means of endosonography. Scand J Gastroenterol 19 (Suppl 94): 60–64, 1984.
11. Strohm WD, Kurtz W, Hagenmüller F, Classen M: Diagnostic efficacy of endoscopic ultrasound tomography in pancreatic cancer and cholestasis. Scand J Gastroenterol 19 (Suppl 102): 18–23, 1984.

12. Tio TL, Tytgat GNJ: Endoscopic ultrasonography in staging local resectability of pancreatic and periampullary malignancy. Scan J Gastroenterol 21 (Suppl 123): 135–142, 1986.

13. Tio TL, Tytgat GNJ: Endoscopic ultrasonography of bile duct malignancy and the preoperative assessment of local resectability. Scand J Gastroenterol 21 (Suppl 123): 151–157, 1986.

14. Yasuda K, Tanaka Y, Fujimoto S, Nakajima M, Kawai K: Use of endoscopic ultrasonography (EUS) on the small pancreatic cancer. Scand J Gastroenterol 19 (Suppl 102): 9–17, 1984.

15. Yasuda K, Nakajima M, Kawai K: Technical aspects of endoscopic ultrasonography of the biliary system. Scand J Gastroenterol 21 (Suppl 123): 143–150, 1986.

16. Yasuda K, Mukai H, Fujimoto S, Nakajima M, Kawai K: Early diagnosis of pancreatic cancer by endoscopic ultrasonography (EUS). Gastrointest Endosc 34: 1–8, 1988.

10

Evaluation of Resectability of Gastrointestinal Tumors

T.L. Tio and G.N.J. Tytgat

Endoscopic ultrasonography (EUS) allows clear visualization of gastrointestinal tumors by directly approaching target lesions via the lumen with a high-frequency ultrasonic beam. EUS allows detailed analysis of all layers of the gastrointestinal wall architecture, presently a shortcoming of conventional diagnostic techniques (1–12). In addition, real-time dynamic properties allow detailed visualization of tumor penetration including extension into surrounding lymph nodes and major vascular structures, thereby improving assessment of resectability. Biliary and pancreatic tumors also can be studied through the stomach and duodenal wall. This chapter describes the accuracy, limitations, and clinical usefulness of EUS in determining the resectability of gastrointestinal malignancy.

ESOPHAGEAL TUMORS

BENIGN TUMORS

Leiomyoma, the most common benign esophageal tumor, is usually seen as a bulging mass covered with smooth mucosa and occasionally with a central ulcer when viewed endoscopically or radiographically. Endoscopic biopsy is rarely helpful in ascertaining the diagnosis and/or in ruling out malignancy. Generally, the submucosal lesion cannot be reached with a standard biopsy forceps except when special techniques are used. With EUS, a leiomyoma appears as a sharply demarcated lesion with a homogeneous echo-structure and echo-pattern under normal-appearing mucosa. Local thickening of the muscularis propria may also be seen. Leiomyomas compress but do not infiltrate into surrounding tissues. A submucosal tumor mass with an inhomogeneous echopattern and less demarcated or bizarrely defined borders is strongly suspicious for a leiomyoblastoma or leiomyosarcoma. Occasionally these contain a central ulcer. Differentiation between a benign and malignant lesion can occasionally be difficult. The presence of suspicious lymph nodes may be helpful in distinguishing the malignant character of the lesion.

MALIGNANT TUMORS

"Early" esophageal carcinoma is visualized as a hypoechoic lesion localized in the mucosa and/or submucosa without penetration into the muscularis propria. There is no evidence of

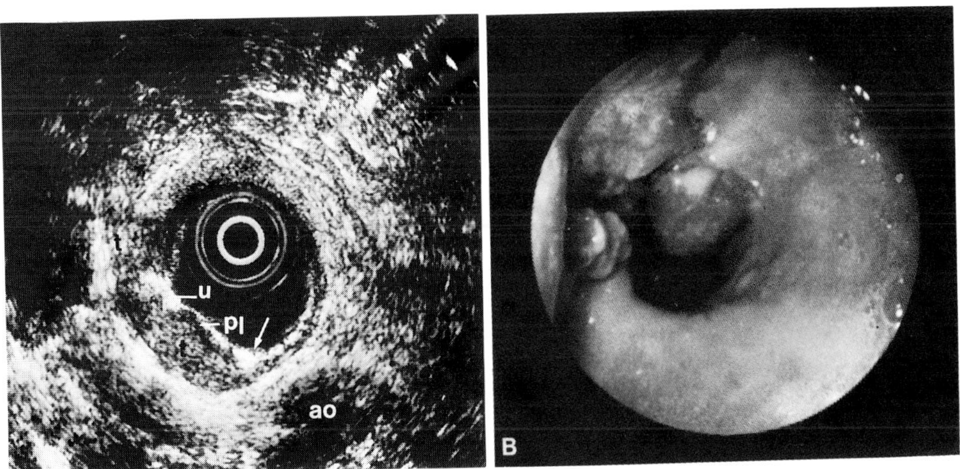

Fig. 10-1. **A.** EUS shows an ulcerative hypoechoic tumor mass (t) with polypoid margins (pl) penetrating into the adventitia and periesophageal fat tissue bordering the aorta (ao). Note the clear transition between the normal and pathologic wall structure (arrow). **B.** Corresponding picture of the polypoid esophageal carcinoma.

Table 10-1. The results of EUS in assessing resectability of esophageal carcinoma.

	EUS–Correct diagnosis	Surgery/histology
Curative resectability	15	18
Palliative resectability	22	26
Nonresectability	10	11

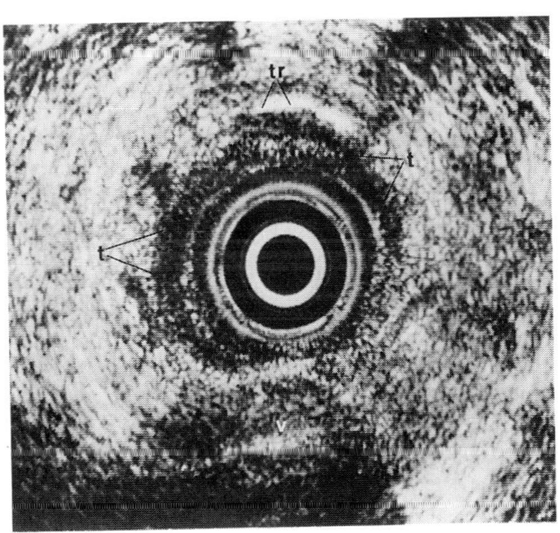

Fig. 10-2. EUS shows a circular hypoechoic transmural tumor mass (t) with deep penetration into the surrounding tissues. The trachea (tr) adjacent to the tumor mass is penetrated. v: vertebra.

adjacent lymph node involvement. In some cases, a benign inflammatory reaction secondary to ulcerative changes of an "early" cancerous lesion may simulate a more deeply infiltrating cancer.

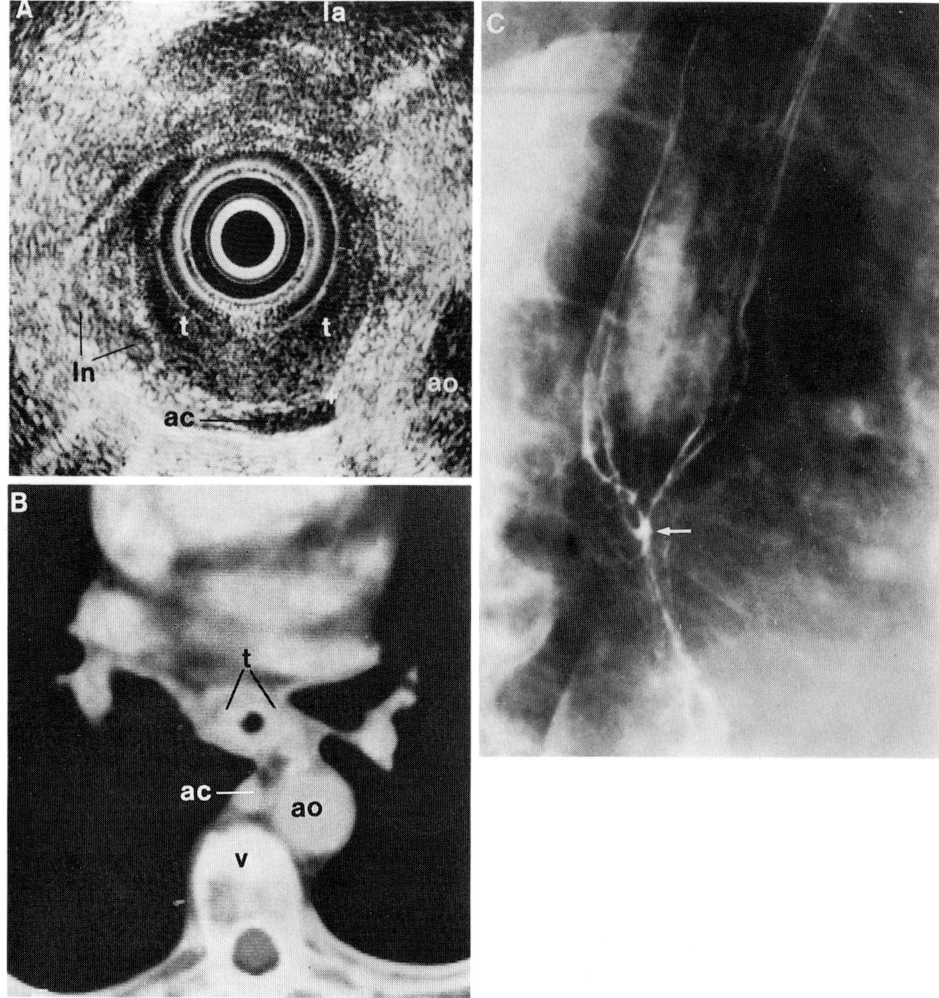

Fig. 10-3. **A.** EUS shows circular transmural hypoechoic structure with deep penetration into the surrounding periesophageal fat tissue bordering the azygos vein. ao: aorta; la: left atrium. **B.** CT reveals thickening of the esophageal wall (t) bordering the azygos vein (ac) and aorta (ao). v: vertrebra. **C.** Corresponding radiogram shows the stenosing esophageal carcinoma (arrow).

In more advanced esophageal cancer, a sonographic diagnosis of local resectability with intention of cure is diagnosed when a well demarcated hypoechoic tumorous lesion is found, without spread through the organ boundaries or to adjacent lymph nodes. Some surgeons claim that regional lymph node involvement does not rule out curative resection. We feel that chances for cure are remote if regional lymph node involvement is found (Fig. 10-1). Resectability is considered palliative in nature when regional and distant lymph node involvement is found in the presence of locally resectable tumor. Some surgeons feel that only distant lymph node metastasis (for example, around the celiac trunk) indicates nonresectability. Evidence of unquestionable nonresectability is diagnosed when there is deep penetration of malignancy into the surrounding tissues, such as the major blood vessels, diaphragm or vertebrae, or adjacent organs, such as the pericardium, tracheobronchial tree, or liver. In such circumstances, the whole tumor cannot be removed from the surrounding tissues or organ

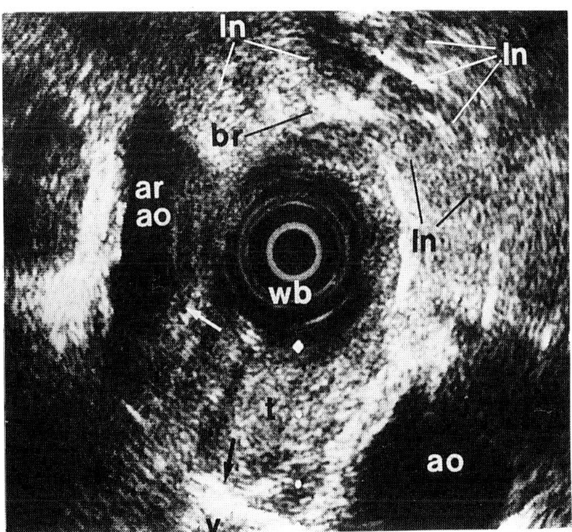

Fig. 10-4. EUS shows a hypoechoic tumor mass with deep penetration, particularly toward the vertebra (v) (black arrow) and aortic arch (ar ao). br: bronchus; ln: lymph nodes; v: vertebra.

Table 10-2. The results of EUS and CT in assessing resectability of esophageal carcinoma with surgery/histology.

	EUS	CT	Surgery/histology
Curative resectability	8	6	10
Palliative resectability	13	7	16
Nonresectability	16	7	18

(11, 12). Data collected in a prospective study and summarized in Table 10-1 support this definition of curative, palliative, and nonresectability.

In cases of extensive deep penetration into or through the adjacent tracheobronchial tree, differentiation between an esophageal and a bronchial or tracheal carcinoma can be difficult (Fig. 10-2); bronchoscopy is helpful in ascertaining the diagnosis. In a prospective study EUS was found to be superior when compared with computed tomography (CT) in determining resectability of esophageal malignancy. The ability to achieve cross-oblique- and longitudinal sections of the tumor and visualizing of the periintestinal lymph nodes even when the diameter was smaller than 5 mm was better than CT scanning (Fig. 10-3). Moreover, the real-time dynamic ultrasonographic properties are superior to the static radiographic device in assessing tumor penetration around or into the adjacent blood vessels (Fig. 10-4). Data collected in Table 10-2 support the superiority of EUS compared with CT in assessing resectability of esophageal carcinoma.

GASTRIC TUMOR

EUS of the stomach is valuable in detecting and staging a gastric neoplasm. When the lesion is found endoscopically, the balloon and/or the lumen can be filled with water to visualize the longitudinal extent and depth of infiltration, together with adjacent lymph node abnormalities.

BENIGN TUMORS

The most important benign lesion is a leiomyoma. Small leiomyomas have a homogeneous echo-pattern and sharply demarcated boundaries. Occasionally, local thickening of the muscularis propria or the muscularis mucosae can be visualized clearly, which helps to ascertain the diagnosis. Large leiomyomas may have an inhomogeneous echo-pattern mostly because of the content of blood vessels, ulcerative or necrotic lesions, or calcification within the tumor masses. The boundaries of lesions are sharply demarcated and compress, but do not penetrate, into the surrounding tissue. Extramural lesions compressing the gastric wall, such as pancreatic pseudocyst, metastatic lymph nodes, fundic varices or aneurysm of the splenic artery, hepatomegaly or splenomegaly, ectopic pancreas, or Ménétrier's disease can be easily ruled out by EUS.

MALIGNANT TUMORS

The most common malignant submucosal lesions are leiomyosarcoma or leiomyoblastoma, which usually reveal an inhomogeneous echo-pattern with the presence of a central ulcer or necrosis. Supplementary findings such as bizarre boundaries and the presence of suspicious lymph nodes may help to ascertain the malignant character of the lesion. However, sharply demarcated boundaries do not exclude malignancy.

The most important and common gastric malignancy is a carcinoma. Early gastric carcinoma is visualized as a hypoechoic echo-pattern localized in the mucosa and/or submucosa without penetration into the muscularis propria with or without adjacent lymph node abnormalities. In contrast, advanced gastric carcinoma is visualized as a hypoechoic intramural lesion with penetration into or through the muscularis propria mostly associated with lymph node abnormalities (Fig. 10-5). In order to assess the accuracy and limitations of EUS in the preoperative assessment of resectability the patients are divided into three groups:

Group 1, Local resectability with intention of curability is diagnosed when EUS visualizes

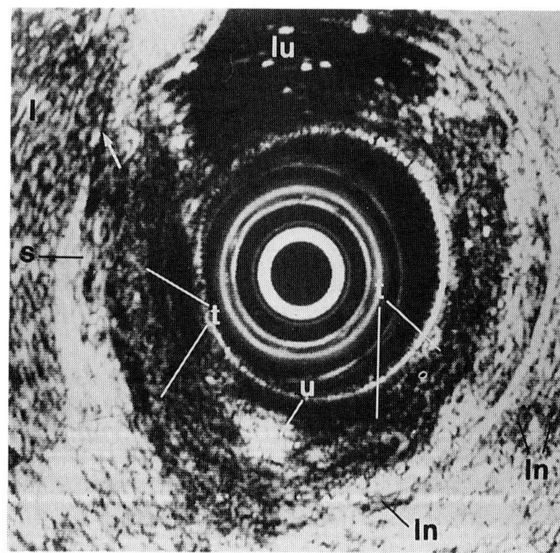

Fig. 10-5. EUS shows a hypoechoic echo-pattern with penetration into the serosal layer (s), with some adjacent lymph nodes (ln) not suspicious of metastatic involvement. Note the unclear boundaries and more hyperechoic echo-pattern of the lymph nodes. u: ulcer; lu: lumen; l: liver.

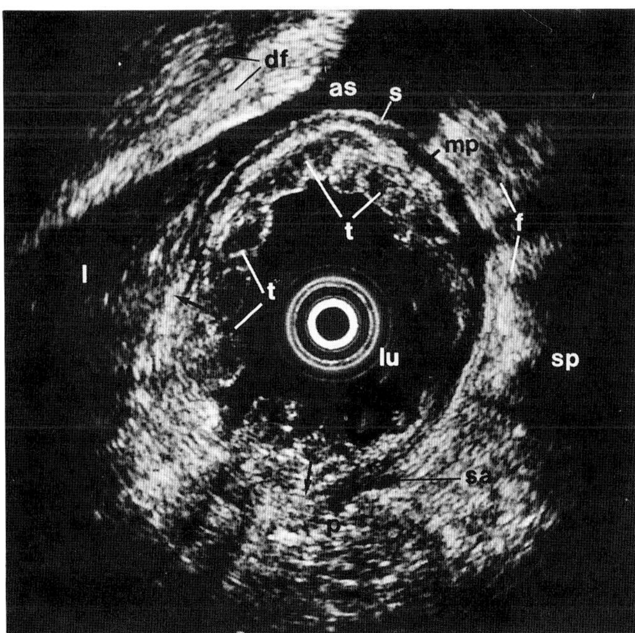

Fig. 10-6. EUS shows diffuse spreading hypoechoic tumor mass (t) in the submucosa with some penetration through the muscularis propria (mp) (arrows). as: ascites; df: diaphragm, l: liver; p: pancreas; s: serosa; sp: spleen; sa: splenic artery.

Table 10-3. The results of EUS in assessing resectability of gastric carcinoma.

	EUS—Correct diagnosis	Surgery/histology
Curative resectability	17	20
Palliative resectability	13	15
Nonresectability	14	17

a clearly demarcated intramural hypoechoic lesion without penetration through the organ boundaries (muscularis propria) with or without adjacent lymph node abnormalities.

Group 2, Palliative resectability is diagnosed when EUS visualizes a sharply demarcated hypoechoic tumor mass without deep penetration into the surrounding tissue and usually with distant lymph node abnormalities.

Group 3, Nonresectability is diagnosed when EUS visualizes deep penetration of a malignancy lesion into the surrounding tissue, for example, major blood vessels, hepatoduodenal ligament, metastases in the greater omentum, or organs such as the pancreas, liver, and colon. In case of diffuse submucosal signet-cell carcinoma of the stomach (linitis plastica) resection usually does not benefit patients. Even if the malignancy were locally resectable, the prognosis is still poor (Fig. 10-6). Data collected in a prospective study and summarized in Table 10-3 support this definition of curative, palliative, and nonresectability.

Non-Hodgkin lymphoma of the stomach is increasingly recognized, major problems often are encountered in staging such lesions. EUS visualizes gastric non-Hodgkin lymphoma as a polypoid, ulcerative, or polypoid ulcerative, and/or diffuse transmural infiltration together with perigastric lymph node abnormalities (10). Occasionally an extensive hypoechoic tumor

Table 10-4. The results of EUS and CT in assessing resectability of gastric carcinoma.

	EUS	CT	Surgery/histology
Curative resectability	17	12	20
Palliative resectability	10	6	13
Nonresectability	13	7	15

mass immediately adjacent to the extensive ulcerative lesion can be identified. Difficulty may arise when giant folds associated with a gastric ulcer simulate a gastric non-Hodgkin lymphoma. This mimicking is caused by the similar transmural hypoechoic echo-pattern, especially when transmural infiltration and an extensive ulcerative lesion are visualized. EUS does not differentiate well between inflammatory changing secondary to ulceration, either in the gastric wall or lymph nodes. Therefore, hypoechoic intramural changes and hypoechoic sharply demarcated lymph nodes adjacent to an ulcerative lesion may be compatible with a benign lesion and do not automatically indicate malignancy. In the near future endosonographic-guided biopsy or cytological puncture may alleviate such a problem. When compared with CT, EUS appears superior in the assessment of resectability of gastric malignancy (Table 10-4).

PANCREATIC TUMORS

BENIGN PANCREATIC LESION MIMICKING PANCREATIC MALIGNANCY

The most common benign pancreatic lesion mimicking pancreatic malignancy is a noncommunicating pancreatic pseudocyst obstructing the main pancreatic duct. By placing the echo probe as close as possible to the obstructive ductular lesion, the distinction between a benign and malignant process can be made. Pancreatic pseudocysts usually are visualized as an anechoic structure with smooth contour, occasionally with some inhomogeneous echo-pattern. In contrast, pancreatic cancer is visualized as a hypoechoic inhomogeneous lesion with polycyclic or bizarre contours, usually associated with suspicious lymph nodes. Groove pancreatitis with irregular abnormality of the common bile duct and/or of the pancreatic duct may strongly mimic pancreatic malignancy on ERCP. EUS allows visualization of the ductular abnormality and determines the presence of a hypoechoic echopattern between the duodenal wall and the pancreas, whereas the pancreatic parenchyma does not suggest malignant transformation.

PANCREATIC CANCER

The transduodenal and transgastric approach allows clear visualization of the pancreas and distal part of the biliary tract. A pancreatic carcinoma is visualized as a hypoechoic sharply or bizarrely demarcated parenchymal echo-pattern, which often appears more hypoechoic than the surrounding tissues. The parenchymal and ductular abnormalities, together with the peripancreatic lymph nodes, can be seen readily. Supplementary findings such as compression of the pancreatic duct, bile duct, or both with prestenotic dilatation corresponding to the ERCP findings of a double duct also help to detect the malignant nature of the lesion.

Resectability for cure is determined by the presence of a hypoechoic pancreatic lesion

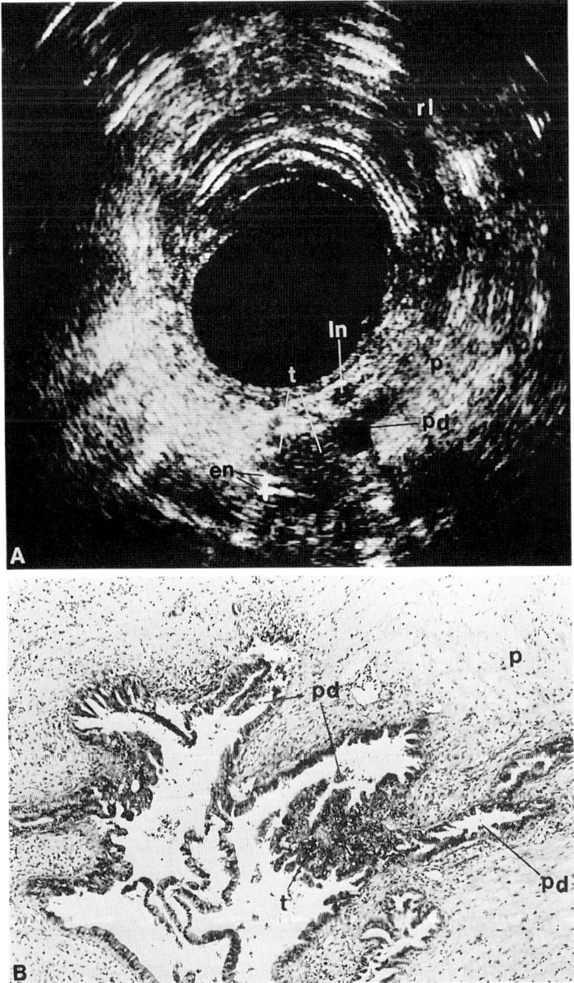

Fig. 10-7. **A.** EUS shows a circumscribed hypoechoic tumor (t) containing the endoprosthesis (en) bordering the pancreatic duct (pd) with a small lymph node (ln) found negative for metastasis by histology. **B.** Corresponding histology of the resection specimen revealing an intraductal carcinoma (t) of the pancreas (p). pd: pancreatic duct.

with a more hypoechoic echo-pattern than the surrounding tissue, together with the absence of penetration into the surrounding blood vessels or adjacent lymph nodes (Fig. 10-7). Intraductular carcinoma, usually multilocated, is visualized as a hypoechoic intraductular lesion originating from the ductular wall. Although the tumors are locally resectable, the prognosis of such a lesion is dubious. A clearly demarcated hypoechoic tumor mass without penetration into the adjacent major blood vessels but with evidence of lymph node involvement indicates the palliative character of the surgical resection. Pancreatic cancer is considered nonresectable when there is deep penetration into the surrounding tissues and/or into the major blood vessels such as the mesenteric artery, celiac trunk, aorta, vena cava, or splenoportal confluens (Fig. 10-8). Visualization of the retroperitoneal area is essential for determining nonresectability. Occasionally an extensive anechoic cavity immediately adjacent to the main lesion can be visualized compatible with a necrotic mass; this also indicates nonresectability (Fig. 10-9).

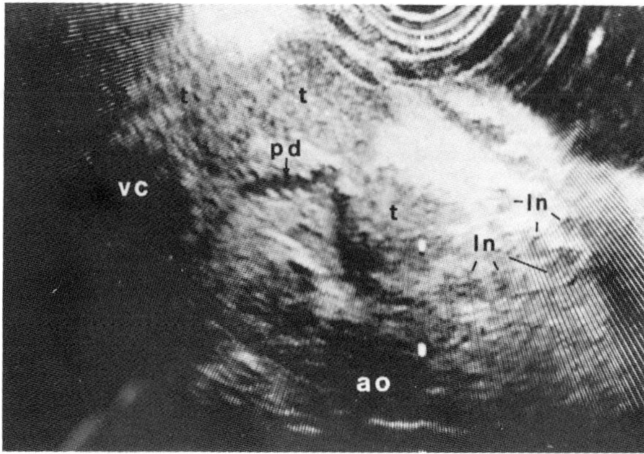

Fig. 10-8. EUS shows a hypoechoic pancreatic tumor mass (t) with clearly demarcated boundaries with compression of the pancreatic duct (pd). Note the retroperitoneal spread of the tumor mass near the aorta (ao) and vena cava (vc). ln: lymph nodes.

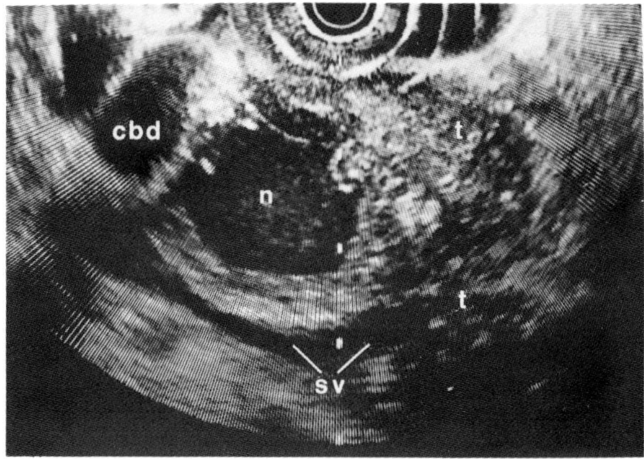

Fig. 10-9. EUS shows an inhomogeneous tumor mass (t) with an adjacent necrotic cavity (n) compressing the common bile duct (cbd). Note the penetration to the splenic vein (sv).

Table 10-5. The results of EUS in assessing resectability of pancreatic carcinoma with surgery/histology.

	EUS	Surgery/histology
Curative resectability	2	3
Palliative resectability	10	11
Nonresectability	5	7

Liver metastasis prohibits curative resection (7, 12). Data collected in Table 10-5 support the value of EUS in defining the curative, palliative, and nonresectability of a pancreatic carcinoma.

PERIPAPILLARY TUMOR

Peripapillary tumor is visualized as a hypoechoic intramural lesion immediately adjacent to

Table 10-6. The results of EUS in assessing resectability of peripapillary carcinoma with surgery/histology.

	EUS—Correct diagnosis	Surgery/histology
Curative resectability	7	9
Palliative resectability	2	3
Nonresectability	2	2

Table 10-7. The results of EUS in assessing resectability of the distal common bile duct carcinoma.

	EUS—Correct diagnosis	Surgery/histology
Curative resectability	4	6
Palliative resectability	8	11
Nonresectability	2	2

the peripapillary common bile duct and/or pancreatic duct. Differentiation between adenomamyomatosis and carcinoma is difficult or impossible, except when evidence of any penetration into or through the muscularis propria is lacking.

Polypoid configuration of the tumor clearly can be seen by rapid filling of the duodenal lumen with water and by approaching the lesion directly with the ultrasonic beam (7, 9, 12). In advanced peripapillary cancer, invasion into the adjacent pancreatic parenchyma clearly can be visualized, which may make the differentiation between pancreatic cancer and peripapillary carcinoma difficult. Data collected in the Table 10-6 support the value of EUS in assessing the curative, palliative and nonresectability of pancreatic cancer.

DISTAL COMMON BILE DUCT LESION

Malignancy in the distal common bile duct is visualized as a polypoid hypoechoic structure originating from the bile duct wall and protruding into the dilated lumen. After insertion of a biliary endoprosthesis, a hypoechoic tumor structure containing a hyperechoic line is characteristic for bile duct malignancy. An endoprosthesis is sometimes a useful guide for localizing the main lesion and does not prohibit accurate visualization of the lesion (Fig. 10-10).

Local resectability with intention of cure can be diagnosed confidently when the tumor is sharply demarcated with or without regional lymph node involvement. A locally resectable tumor with multiple regional and distant suspicious lymph nodes suggests the palliative character of the resection. Bile duct malignancy with deep penetration into the adjacent pancreas often can cause difficulties with respect to differentiation from a pancreatic carcinoma. The presence of a pancreatic duct abnormality is more characteristic for pancreatic carcinoma than for bile duct malignancy. Evidence of nonresectability can be ascertained based on penetration of tumor into the adjacent major blood vessels, such as the hepatic artery, portal vein, celiac trunk, aorta, or vena cava, and/or metastasis to the liver (7, 12). The topographic anatomical relationship between the papilla of Vater, distal common bile duct, and pancreatic duct may at times make exact identification of the origin of tumor difficult. The possibility for an endosonographically-guided puncture will enhance further the value of EUS. Data collected in Table 10-7, support the value of EUS in defining the curative, palliative and nonresectability of a common bile duct carcinoma.

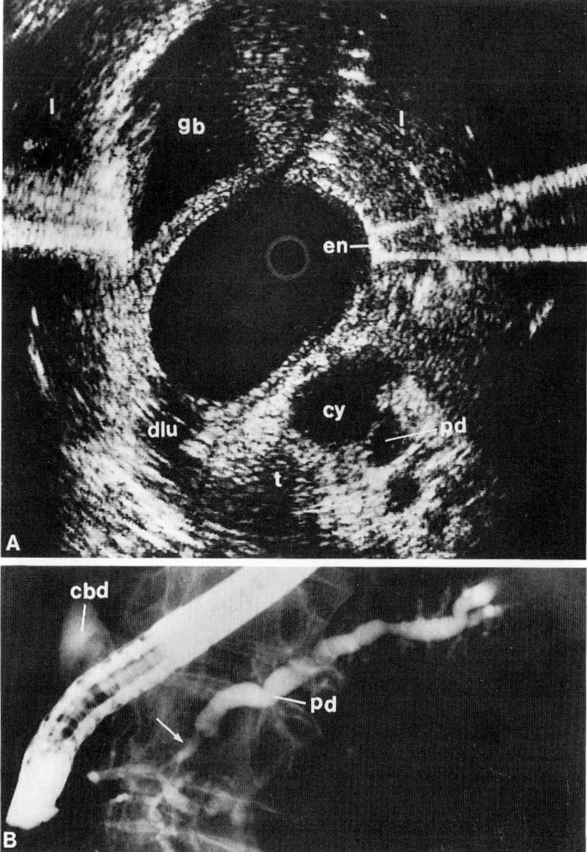

Fig. 10-10. **A**. EUS shows a circumscribed hypoechoic tumor (t) with adjacent cystic lesions (cy) compressing the pancreatic duct (pd). dlu: duodenal lumen; l: liver; en: biliary endoprosthesis; gb: gallbladder. **B**. Corresponding ERCP shows the dilated common bile duct (cbd) and some irregularity of the adjacent pancreatic duct (arrow). pd: pancreatic duct.

TUMOR OF THE HEPATOBILIARY BIFURCATION (KLATSKIN TUMOR)

The biliary tree can be recognized by withdrawing the instrument slowly from the area of the papilla of Vater and using the typical localization of the common bile duct immediately adjacent to the duodenal wall as a landmark. From the apical bulbar scanning position, the liver hilum and gallbladder can be visualized. The confluence of the hepatic duct in the porta hepatis usually is readily recognizable. A malignancy usually is visualized as a hypoechoic intraductular structure localized immediately adjacent to the bifurcation of the bile duct together with dilatation of the intrahepatic ducts and a normal caliber distal common bile duct. A clearly demarcated intraductal lesion localized only in one liver lobe without penetration into the adjacent liver and the portal vein indicates local resectability with intention of cure. A hypoechoic tumor mass extending into both adjacent liver lobes with local penetration into the portal vein, along with multiple suspicious lymph nodes, strongly suggests the palliative nature of the procedure. Deep penetration of a hypoechoic tumor mass into the adjacent major blood vessels, such as the portal vein, hepatic artery, or multiple liver metastasis, is considered

Table 10-8. The results of EUS in assessing resectability of a Klatskin tumor with histology of the resection specimens.

	EUS—Correct diagnosis	Surgery/histology
Curative resectability	2	3
Palliative resectability	12	12

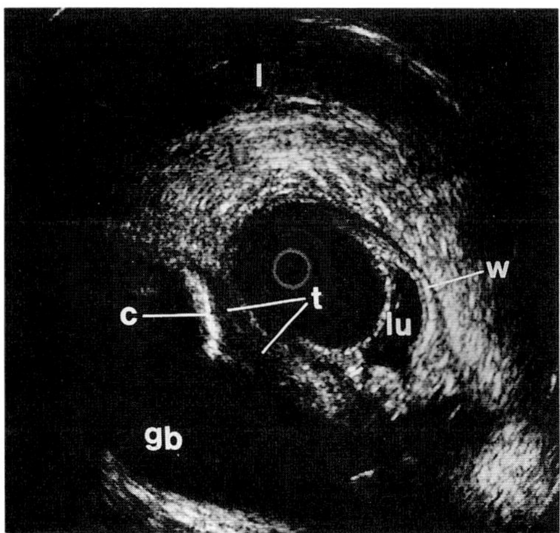

Fig. 10-11. EUS shows a hypoechoic tumor mass (t) in the wall of the gallbladder (gb) with some penetration near the adjacent duodenal lumen (lu). w: normal duodenal wall on the contralateral side; c: concrement in the gallbladder; l: right lobe of the liver.

nonresectable (7, 12). Data collected in Table 10-8 support the value of EUS in defining the curative and palliative resection of a Klatskin tumor. Follow-up investigation after liver resection is accurate and essential because both lymph node abnormality and/or intraductular tumor recurrence can readily be visualized. This is of utmost improtance since ERCP usually is technically impossible after hepaticojejunostomy. Conventional ultrasonography and CT are considerably less accurate in detecting such recurrent malignancies.

GALLBLADDER MALIGNANCY

Carcinoma of the gallbladder is visualized as a hypoechoic polypoid tumor structure originating from the wall or protruding into the cavity of the gallbladder (Fig. 10-11). In an advanced stage, tumor extension along the hepatic duct into the hepatobiliary bifurcation can be recognized. In such cases, differentiation between a Klatskin tumor and a gallbladder carcinoma often is difficult or impossible. Hydrops of the gallbladder due to primary cholangiocarcinoma can be readily differentiated from concrements in the cystic duct, such as seen in the Mirrizzi syndrome. Evidence of nonresectability is based on deep penetration of the malignancy into the surrounding tissues or the adjacent liver parenchyma. An extensive hypoechoic tumor mass of the gallbaldder with penetration into the adjacent gastroduodenal wall with or without lymph node metastases in the pancreatic head may mimic the presence of pancreatic cancer or groove pancreatitis. However, supplementary findings such as compression of the pancreatic duct with prestenotic dilatation of both the pancreatic duct and common bile duct, compatible with a double duct lesion found by ERCP, may help to distinguish malignancy in the gallbladder from cancer of the pancreas.   An endosonographically-guided cytological puncture or biopsy may ascertain the malignant nature of such lesions.

References

1. Caletti G, Bolondi L, Brocchi P, et al.: Staging of gastric cancer by means of endoscopic ultrasono-graphy (abstr). Gastroenterology 84: 13866, 1983.
2. Di Magno EP, Regan PT, Clain JE, James EM, Buxton JL: Human endoscopic ultrasonography. Gastroenterology 83: 824–829, 1982.
3. Heyder N, Lutz H, Lux G: Ultraschalldiagnostik via Gastroskop. Ultraschall Med 4: 84–93, 1983.
4. Lux G, Heyder N, Demling L: Endoscopic ultrasonography—Technique, orientation and diagnostic possibilities. Endoscopy 4: 220–225, 1982.
5. Scand J Gastroenterol 19 (Suppl 102): 5–37, 1984.
6. Scand J Gastroenterol 19 (Suppl 94): 1–106, 1984.
7. Scand J Gastroenterol 21 (Suppl 123): 1–169, 1986.
8. Strohm WD, Classen M: Endosonographie mit einem Gastrofiberskop. Ultraschall Med 5: 84–93, 1984.
9. Tio TL, Tytgat GNJ: Endoscopic ultrasonography in the assessment of intra- or transmural infiltra-tion of tumours in the oesophagus, stomach and papilla of Vater and in the detection of extraoeso-phageal lesions. Endoscopy 4: 220–225, 1984.
10. Tio TL, den Hartog Jager FCA, Tytgat GNJ: Endoscopic ultrasonogaphy of non-Hodgkin lymphoma of the stomach. Gastroenterology 91: 401–408, 1986.
11. Tio TL, den Hartog Jager FCA, Tytgat GNJ: The role of endoscopic ultrasonography in assessing local resectability of oesophagogastric malignancies. Scand J Gastroenterol 21 (Suppl 123): 78–86, 1986.
12. Tio TL, Tytgat GNJ: Atlas of Transintestinal Ultrasonography. Mur Kostverloren BV, Aalsmeer, The Netherlands, 1986.

11

Laparoscopic Sonography in Differential Diagnosis of Liver Diseases

Morimichi Fukuda and Satoaki Mima

Peritoneoscopy is an invasive technique, yet it is an extremely precise diagnostic tool for investigating intraperitoneal organs such as the liver, pancreas, and gallbladder. Precise diagnostic information on liver, either diffuse or localized, can be obtained only by direct visual assessment of the disease expressed on the surface of the liver along with a histologic examination of tissue specimen. Accurate diagnosis of diffuse liver disease including classification and staging of various types of chronic hepatitis, liver cirrhosis, and fatty liver can be made only by this technique. On the other hand, ultrasonic examination of soft tissues, especially of the liver, has facilitated noninvasive detection of benign and malignant mass lesions, differentiation between solid and cystic lesions, and detection of abscess formation. The ability of this method to detect mass lesions in the liver improved markedly since the introduction of real-time ultrasound (10, 12, 13).

The combination of laparoscopic sonography and a sonolaparoscope, equipped with either a mechanical scanner or electronic linear-array probe, is far superior to conventional ultrasound (7, 8). In this chapter, we describe further studies of the use of radial scanning sonolaparoscope in liver disease and our recent results on the use of the new sonolaparoscope equipped with a linear-array 7.5 MHz probe.

EQUIPMENT

To carry out our study we used the prototype 3 sonolaparoscope, Olympus LPS-UM1/EUM1, manufactured by Olympus Optical Co., Tokyo, Japan (Fig. 11-1). The equipment comprises a regular laparoscope with a scanning compartment in which a small transducer (0.7 cm, 10 MHz) is placed at the tip of the scanning chamber of the scope. The scope is housed with an ultrasonic mirror that rotates by a DC motor placed at the hand-grip portion of the scope.

The mechanical radial scanning provides a 180° radial scan sonogram perpendicular to the axis of the scope and is displayed on a cathode ray tube (CRT) screen, at the frame rate of 30 per second. We measured the size and distance of the objects imaged on the CRT screen by an electronic caliper. An image field can be rotated up to 45° in each direction for a total scan field of 270°. The equipment also can be used interchangeably with a regular laparoscope during a peritoneoscopy, through the same trocar, thus reducing intervention to the patient.

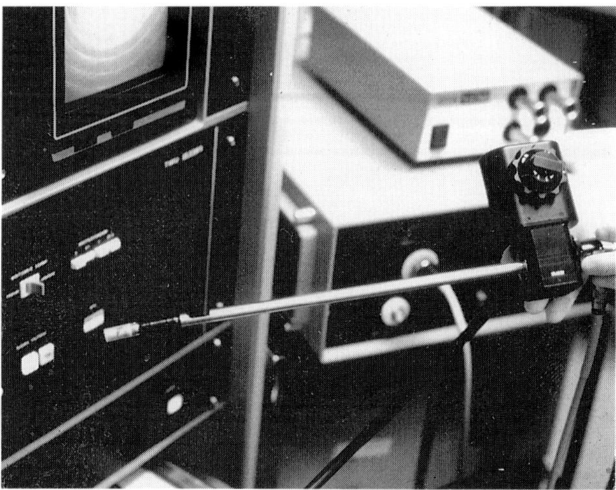

Fig. 11-1. Sonolaparoscope, prototype 3. A fixed transducer, disc type, 7.5 or 10 MHz in frequency, 7 mm in diameter is housed in a scanning compartment. Scanning is carried out by rotating an ultrasonic mirror in the scanning compartment.

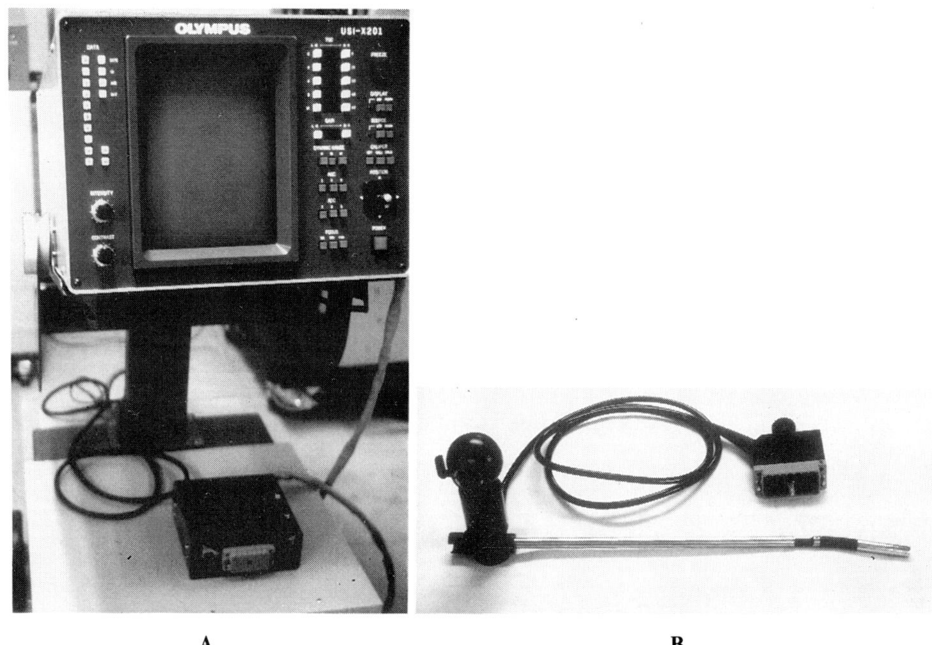

A   B

Fig. 11-2. Electronic sonolaparoscope prototype 1 (**A**) with a linear array probe (**B**) of 7.5 MHz made by Olympus Optical Co., Tokyo.

OLYMPUS ELECTRONIC LINEAR ARRAY SONOLAPAROSCOPE, PROTOTYPE 1

The Olympus electronic linear-array sonolaparoscope recently has become available for investigating its possible clinical application in diagnosing various liver diseases. The equipment consists of an image developing unit and a laparoscope mounted with the linear-array scanner, 7.5 MHz, 4 cm long, with a scanning width of 3.5 cm × 7 cm. The scanning compartment rotates 90° to each side. Its flat surface corresponds to the emission port of sonic waves from the transducer (Fig. 11-2).

Manipulation of the scope is the same as the mechanical scanner: one uses the optical system in the scope to guide its tip. The scope is sterilized in a formalin gas chamber at least 24 hours before each examination.

METHOD

After routine laparoscopic examination, the sonolaparoscope is introduced into the abdominal cavity through the same trocar and scanning head, which is bent approximately 90° toward the axis of the scope. This brings the liver into view of the scope. Scanning begins by pressing a switch on the front panel of the imaging unit; tomographic images are displayed on the viewing screen as real-time CRT images. The image can either be photographed directly from the screen or recorded on video cassette for further evaluation. The images also may be recorded at a real-time dynamic scanning made or at times of image-freezing. The latter method is preferred over simple real-time recording because of the rapid movement of targets during examination.

Scanning by the sonolaparoscope equipped with a linear-array probe is essentially the same as described above, except the images displayed are 3.5 × 7 cm rather than the radial scan field.

SUBJECTS

From October 1980 to September 1985, 195 laparoscopic ultrasound examinations were performed on 183 cases suffering from various intraabdominal disorders. Another series of patients comprising 35 cases recently were examined with the linear-array sonolaparoscope. Results of the latter series were positive, in view of the ease of operation and virtually no mechanical complications (which have been experienced frequently with the former type of sonolaparoscope).

SONOLAPAROSCOPIC IMAGE OF THE LIVER

High quality ultrasonic images were obtained by sonolaparoscopic examination, as indicated earlier (8). Sonographic texture of liver parenchyma was finer than those obtained by routine sonography performed on the body surface. The portal vein branches of the normal liver showed smooth tapering, whereas cirrhotic liver invariably displayed dilatation of the tributaries of the portal vein system with a slightly jagged, irregular appearance to its periphery. In advanced liver cirrhosis, several sonographic features were demonstrated, such as the marked degrees of parenchymal atrophy, as evidenced by marked shrinkage of a cross-sectional area of the hepatic lobe, macronodular change of liver parenchyma (Fig. 11-3), and thickening of periportal fat tissues as thick echogenic layers surrounding the portal vein stems. However, in micronodular cirrhosis (frequently found in advanced alcoholics), the sonolaparoscopic

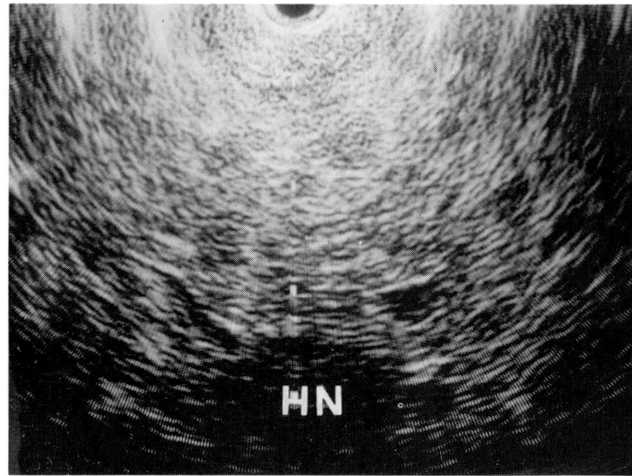

Fig. 11-3. A sonogram of macronodular liver cirrhosis by the radial scan sonolaparoscope. The large hypoechoic nodule (HN) was the hyperplastic nodule confirmed by surgical operation.

Table 11-1. Diagnostic accuracy of sonolaparoscopy (Olympus LPS-UM1/EUM1).

Disease	No. of Cases	True Positive	False Negative
Hepatocellular carcinoma	50	41 (82%)	9 (18%)*
Hemangioma	17	16 (94%)	1 (6%)
Cholangiocellular carcinoma	2	2	0
Liver cyst	7	7	0
Multiple biliary hamartoma	3	3	0
Focal nodular hyperplasia	2	2	0
Echinococcosis	1	1	0
Tuberculoma	1	1	0
Adenomatous hyperplasia	1	1	0

* Among 9 cases of HCC not visualized, 7 were owing to deep location of tumors for detection, whereas in the remaining two cases failure was owing to too superficial location of the small isoechoic mass.

image did not differ much from normal patients unless large regenerative nodules were formed.

IMAGING CAPABILITY OF SONOLAPAROSCOPY

Among 160 cases examined by the sonolaparoscope LPS-UM1, 84 cases were suspected of liver tumors after x-ray CT, routine ultrasound, nuclear imaging, and celiac angiography diagnoses were made. The success rate of comparable diagnosis in sonolaparoscopic imaging of the lesions is shown in Table 11-1.

Among various hepatic lesions examined, 41 cases (82%) with hepatocellular carcinoma (HCC) were successfully visualized, whereas 9 cases escaped detection: either the mass was too deep to be imaged or the isoechogenicity of the mass was too superficial for adequate visualization. Only one case of hemangioma escaped detection.

CHARACTERISTICS OF SONOGRAPHIC IMAGES

Hemangioma

Hepatic hemangioma displays characteristic echo-patterns: diffusely hyperechoic, hypoechoic, or marginal echo-pattern types (Fig. 11-4). However, if the tumor size is 1 cm or so in diameter, differentiation between hemangioma from HCC or other metastatic tumors of similar sizes often becomes difficult.

Ultrasonic examination by sonolaparoscopy discloses characteristic features of hemangioma, such as the absence of a hypoechoic halo specific to hepatoma nodules, uniform hyperechogenicity of the mass, and septal structure coinciding to vessel structure in the mass.

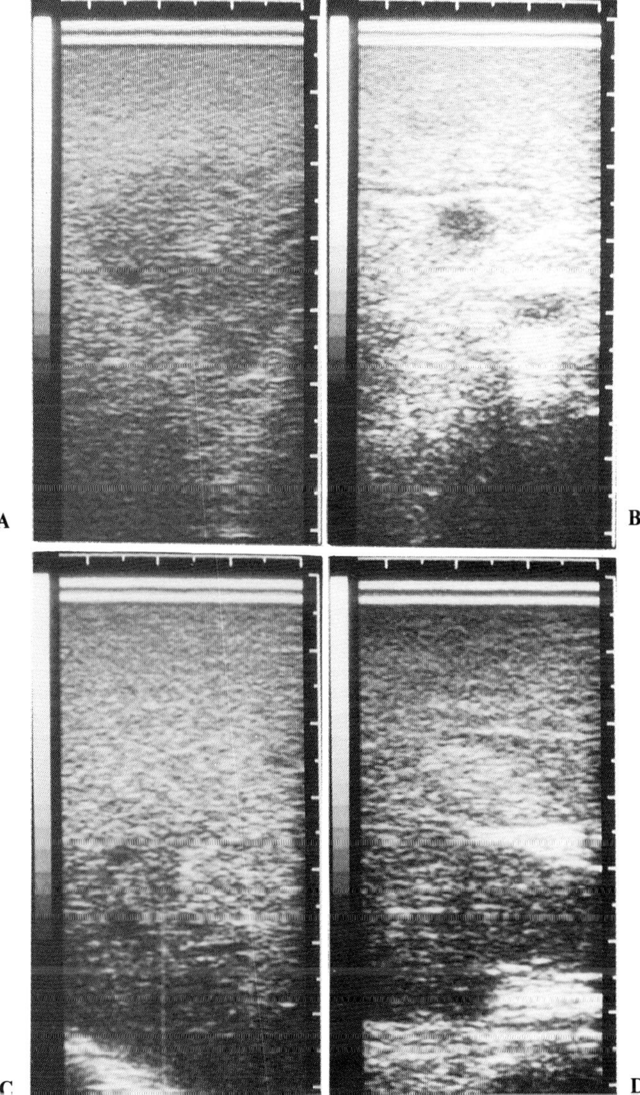

Fig. 11-4. Sonograms of four cases of hemangioma by the linear-array sonolaparoscope.

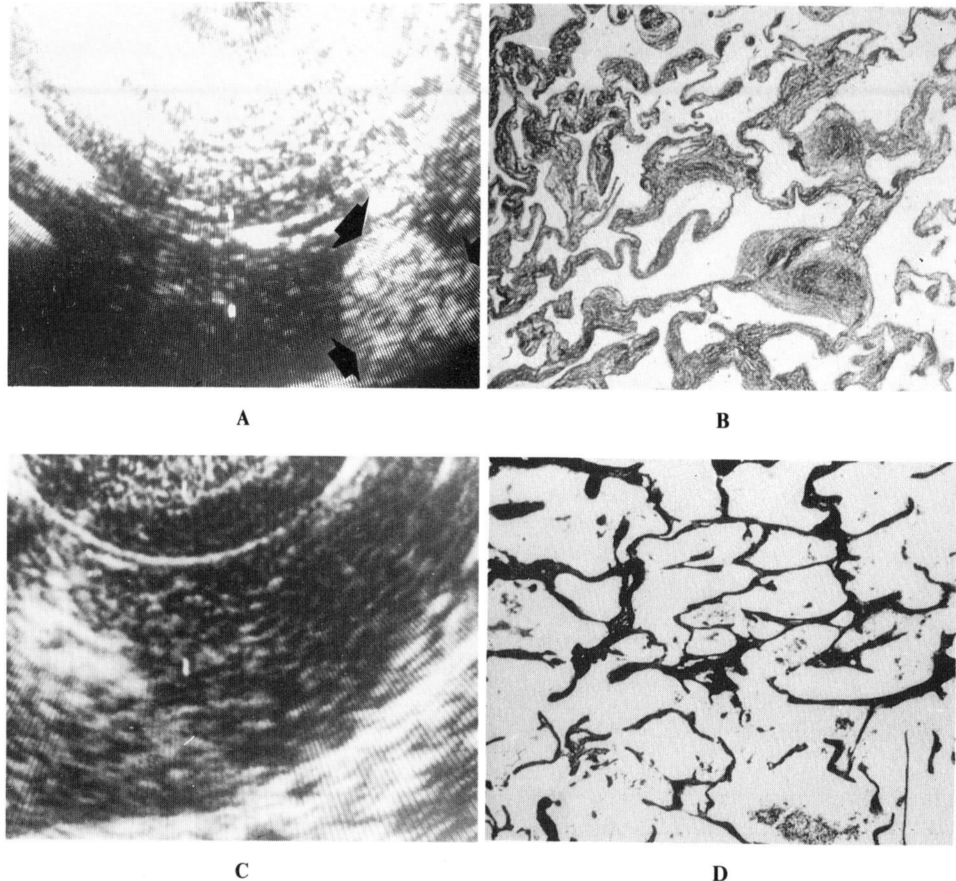

Fig. 11-5. Sonograms of hepatic hemangioma with hyperechoic (**A**) and hypoechoic (**C**) patterns by sono-laparoscopy and corresponding histology (**B, D**) by HE staining.

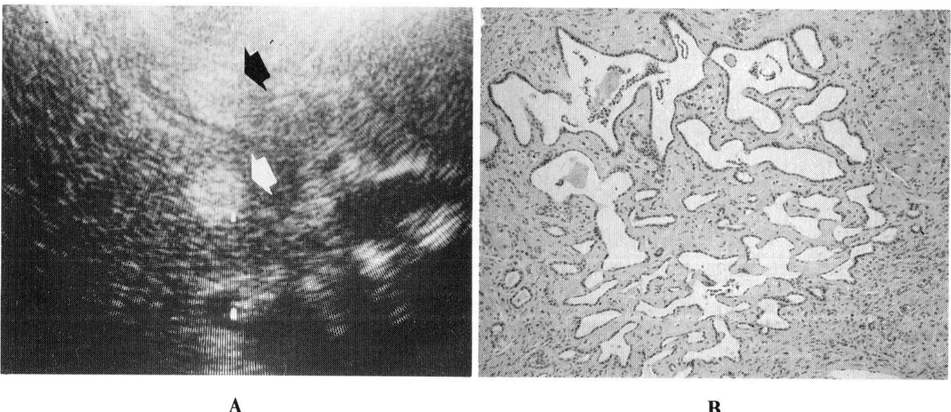

Fig. 11-6. A sonogram of multiple biliary hamartoma of the liver (arrow) with corresponding histology (**B**).

Histopathological examination shows consistent correlation between echogenicity of hemangiomata by sonolaparoscopy and histological findings. The hypoechoic hemangioma generally exhibits thinning of sinusoidal walls to fewer than 200 microns thick, whereas the reverse is true in the hyperechoic hemangioma (Fig. 11-5).

Multiple Biliary Hamartoma

Multiple biliary hamartoma is a rare benign disease of the liver. It is not difficult to diagnose this disease endoscopically, if the characteristic findings, scattered small whitish spots and small elevations with dark greenish discoloration, are present. In routine ultrasound examination, this disease shows a peculiar echo-pattern, the scattered tiny echogenic spots with or without the comet sign. Sonolaparoscopic examination discloses a characteristic echo-pattern such as hyperechoic spots with spoke-in-wheel type appearance. Two cases were examined in our study. Echo-pattern and histological findings are shown in Fig. 11-6.

Hepatocellular Carcinoma

Hepatocellular carcinoma (HCC) in its early stage appears by real-time ultrasound as a small hypoechoic mass. It appears more frequently as a hyperechoic mass when the tumor is more than 3 cm in diameter. The most probable cause for such heterogeneity is fatty metamorphosis of the tumor tissue and, in some cases perhaps, widening of sinusoidal spaces similar to hemangioma or necrosis in the tumor tissue.

In sonolaparoscopy, most of the small liver cancers show slightly increased echo-intensity without any noticeable degree of fatty loading or necrosis (Fig. 11-7). In a few cases, a fine mosaic echo-pattern was noticed in the hepatoma nodule. In a small percentage of cases, early liver cancer may exhibit the bright echo-pattern, resembling those of hepatic hemangioma; the pattern is mainly caused by fatty loading of the tumor tissues (Fig. 11-8).

HCC sometimes exhibits an isoechoic appearance without the distinct halo formation in

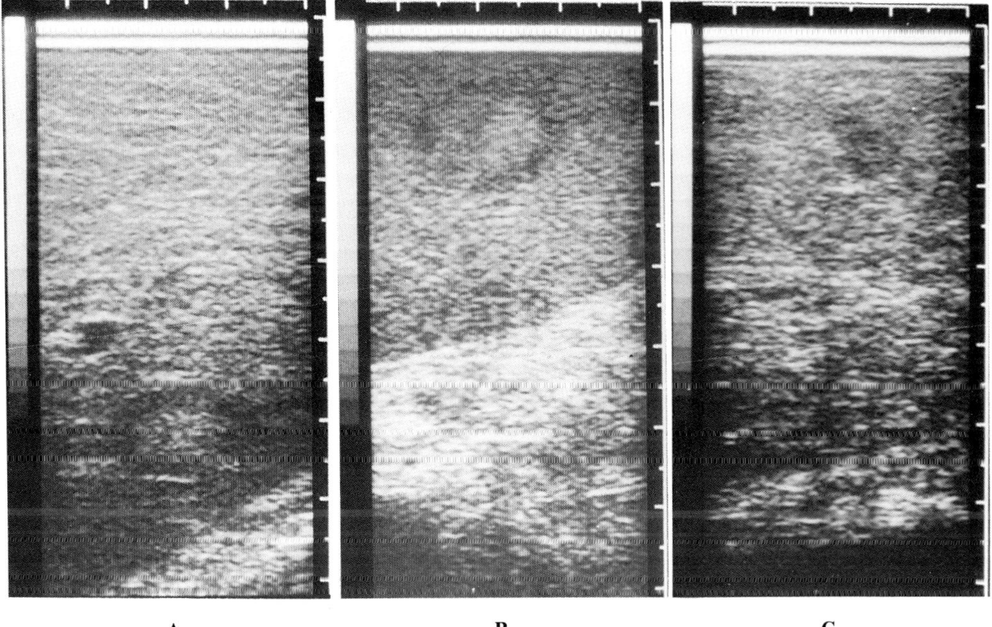

A   B   C

Fig. 11-7. Sonograms of three cases with small HCC by electronic sonolaparoscopy.

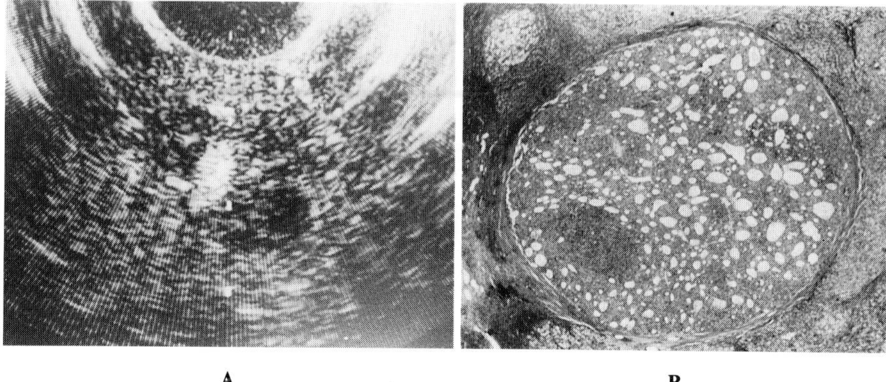

A   B

Fig. 11-8. A radial scan ultrasonogram (**A**) of HCC with bright echo-pattern with histology specimen (**B**. HE staining).

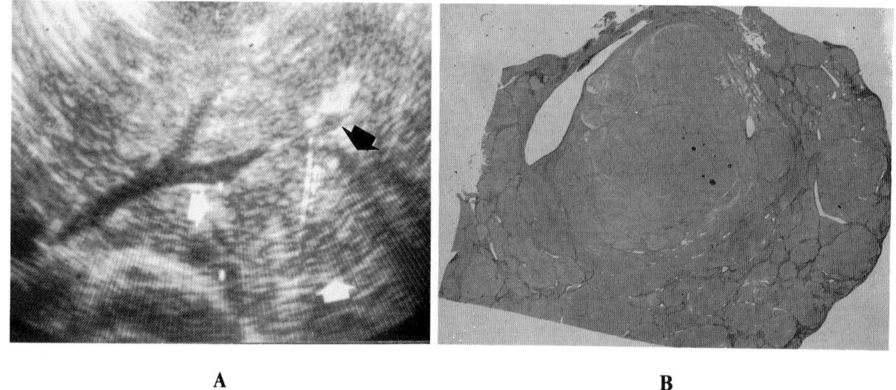

A   B

Fig. 11-9. A radial scan ultrasonogram (**A**) of isoechoic HCC (arrow) in the left lobe of the liver with histology specimen (**B**. HE staining).

its periphery.   Detection and differentiation of HCC are difficult on sonolaparoscopic observation; careful observation of tissue movement and the loss of pulsatile movement owing to expansive growth of the malignant tumor may be the only definite sign to express the nature of the mass.   Figure 11-9 is an example of such a case of HCC observed in a 47-year-old female patient with concomitant chronic hepatitis.   Owing to an increased level of alpha-fetoprotein, the patient was examined by ultrasound, which disclosed a small hypoechoic mass in the left lobe of the liver.   X-ray CT with the bolus injection method displayed a small tumor mass at the same location with initial intense staining.   Sonolaparoscopic examination disclosed an isoechogenic mass with less distinct contours at the posterior part of the left lobe of the liver. Surgical resection was performed, revealing a 1.7 × 1.5 × 1.5 cm liver cancer with a medium degree of fibrosis and nodule formation.   Histological classification was Edmondson type II to III and no fat deposition was observed (Fig. 11-9).

Cholangiocellular Carcinoma of the Liver
Primary hepatic cholangiocellular carcinoma is encountered less frequently than HCC in routine practice.   Certain features are noted in both x-ray CT and ultrasound.   It occurs gen-

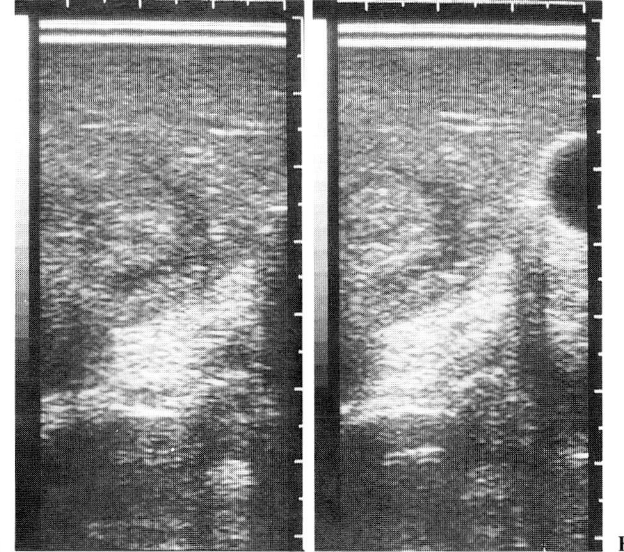

Fig. 11-10. Sonograms of cholangiocellular carcinoma of the liver obatined by the electronic laparoscope.

erally close to the hepatic hilum, and a bizzare-shaped mass with occluded intrahepatic bile ducts in the periphery are the specific features of the mass. The mass may be accompanied by central liquefaction owing to the central necrosis of the mass. Fig. 11-10 shows a sonogram obtained by sonolaparoscopy employing the scope equipped with the linear-array probe. An isoechogenic tumor mass circumscribed by a slightly thicker hypoechoic zone with irregular boundary was identified in the hilar region of the liver. Histological examination after extirpation of the mass confirmed the diagnosis.

Focal Nodular Hyperplasia

Focal nodular hyperplasia (FNH) shows hypoechoic mass formation in the liver parenchyma by ultrasound. The characteristic feature is the presence of central scarring with regenerative change surrounding the scar. The cause of the disease is unknown.

Fig. 11-11 demonstrates a typical case of FNH. The patient was discovered during the mass survey for liver cancer by ultrasound with serum battery tests, and an initial finding was a small, poorly demarcated hypoechoic nodule in the right lobe of the liver. No abnormality was checked by either x-ray CT or angiography. Sonolaparoscopy showed the characteristic echopattern of the ground glass appearance. Resection of the mass was performed, and histological diagnosis was typical FNH with characteristic central scarring. Similar findings were obtained from another male patient in whom we uncovered a small nodular mass in the liver which showed a similar echo pattern. Histological findings of the mass coincided with FNH (Fig. 11-12).

Hyperplasia

Among the benign lesions in the liver to be differentiated from HCC, adenomatous hyperplasia most closely resembles HCC. In fact, the lesion often is considered as one of the precancerous lesions of primary liver cancer.

A 63-year-old man was hospitalized because of chronic hepatitis of non-A, non-B type and an increased level of alpha-fetoprotein. He subsequently underwent a series of diagnostic

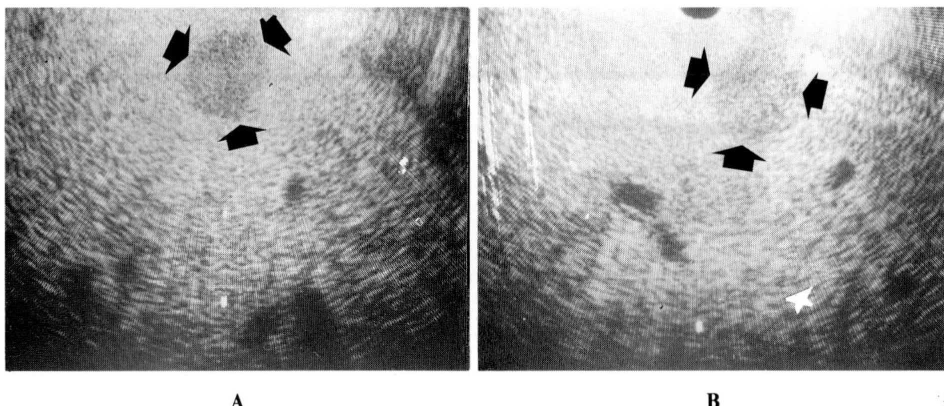

A   B

Fig. 11-11.   Sonograms of a case with FNH.   Note characteristic ground glass appearance of the mass (arrow).

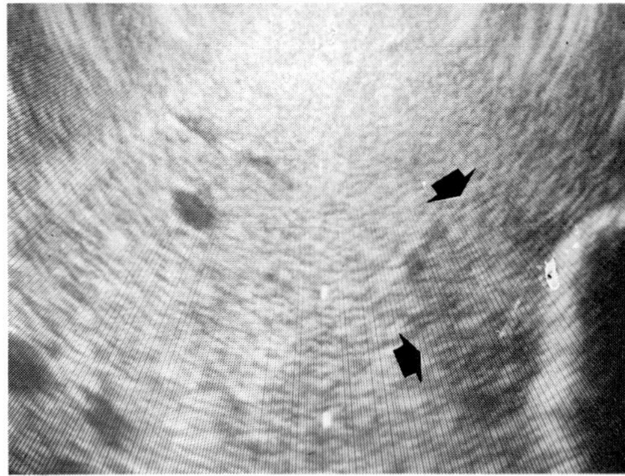

Fig. 11-12.   Sonogram of FNH with peculiar echo-pattern with the central stellate configuration (arrows).

imaging.   Despite the presence of a hypoechoic mass lesion in the right lobe of the liver, the patient failed to show any abnormality on x-ray examination.   By superselective angiography via A. hepatica propria, we found a hypovascular area containing tiny hypervascular spots approximately 3 cm in diameter.   Sonolaparoscopy disclosed the presence of a hypoechoic nodule and a small hemangioma with increased echoegenicity.   In the hypoechoic mass, there were two small echogenic spots 5 and 2 mm in diameter (Fig. 11-13).   The patient subsequently underwent segmental resection of a portion of the right lobe of the liver.   Histopathological examination revealed one 8 mm diameter hemangioma and two hyperplastic nodules, 0.6 cm and 2.2 × 1.8 cm.   In the larger hyperplastic nodule, two tiny hepatocellular carcinomas were found with diameters of 0.7 cm and 0.3 cm (Fig. 11-13).

Solitary Tuberculoma
Granulomatous lesions in the liver, especially tuberculous granulomata, are rare.   Fig. 11-14 demonstrates a peculiar feature of the tuberculous granulomata: In this case, routine real-time ultrasonic examination and sonolaparoscopy showed an echo-pattern similar to a hypoechoic nodule.   Sonolaparoscopy disclosed an irregular-shaped hypoechoic nodule with a well-circumscribed border without any sign of expansiveness.   Histological examination disclosed a sharply demarcated lesion of coagulation necrosis characteristic of tuberculous granulomata.

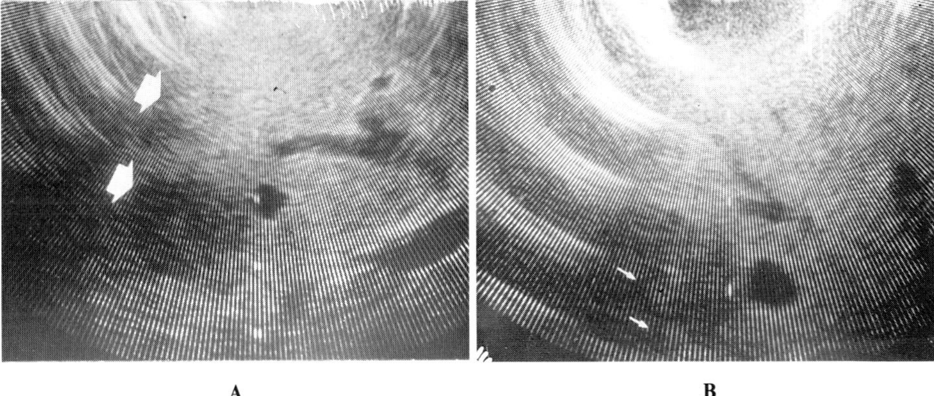

A   B

Fig. 11-13. Sonograms of parenchymatous hyperplasia of the liver. Sonograms were recorded by 10 MHz radial scan sonolaparoscope. Large arrows (**A**) indicate small hemangioma and parenchymatous hyperplasia and two small arrows (**B**) indicate minute HCC in the nodule.

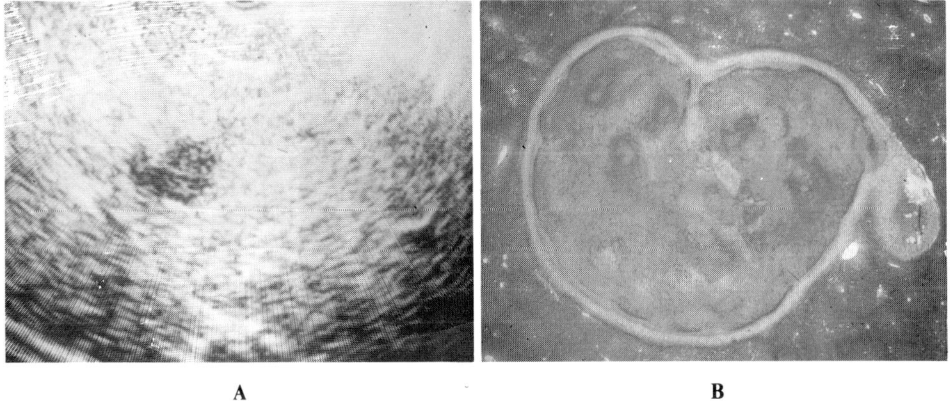

A   B

Fig. 11-14. Sonogram (**A**) of tuberculous granuloma of the liver with hitology finding (**B**) stained by HE stain.

DISCUSSION

Rapid screening of intrahepatic mass lesions is well facilitated by real-time ultrasound. This technique is noninvasive and economic, but it is hampered by the lack of specific histopathological diagnosis and by individual dependence of the diagnostic accuracy. Laparoscopy allows precise diagnosis of the liver, gallbladder, and other intraabdominal organs based on specific findings demonstrated on the peritoneal surface of respective organs (2). Its main shortcoming is inability to diagnose hidden lesions in the organ. To overcome these defects, high-resolution ultrasonography by sonolaparoscopy was attempted (1, 7, 8, 11, 14).

Direct scanning of the liver by an endoprobe attached to a peritoneoscope was not performed until recently because of the lack of a high-frequency transducer and electronic technology available. The first report on the sonolaparoscope to use a rotating mechanical transducer was in 1981(6); further details were described subsequently (8). Apparatus similar to the linear-array transducer but with a lower frequency (5 MHz) was introduced simultaneously (14) with the sonolaparoscope. As mentioned earlier, combined use of the ultrasonic scanner in the peritoneoscopy has a marked advantage over the use of either technique alone. The sonolaparoscopic examination furnishes sonograms with increased spatial and contrast resolution and helps to establish precise diagnosis of diseases of intraabdominal organs.

The advantages of high-frequency transducers were not recognized in the past. As shown in the cases presented above, laparoscopic sonography by a 10 MHz transducer reflected histopathological findings regarding size and internal structures of mass lesions. Laparoscopic sonography enables recognition of the differences between hepatic hemangioma and HCC based on sonographic features such as the shape, internal ultrasonic textures, presence or absence of boundary echoes, mosaic echo-pattern in HCC nodules, presence or absence of posterior echo enhancement, and invasion into the intrahepatic vessels. B-mode echo-pattern analysis by sonolaparoscopy may not be the sole characterization of the tumor mass in question; however, the high resolution of the images obtained by this technique surpasses the other imaging modalities currently available.

It is still to be determined which sonolaparoscope—linear array or mechanical radial scanner—is adequate for standard examination. Our experience and that of others favors the latter because of its superior imaging capability. A disadvantage to this method, however, is the anticipated mechanical troubles inherent in such a system. Although the images obtained by the linear-array sonolaparoscope are limited by the slightly inferior resolution and narrower scan field compared with the mechanical radial scanner, the linear-array version may surpass the mechanical radial scanner because of the lack of mechanical dysfunction and sensitivity to the distant portions of large organs. The linear-array version also can be used for ultrasound-guided biopsy. This technique is described by Boenhof et al., and Frank et al., using the sonolaparoscope equipped with a linear-array scanner (3-5).

The equipment currently available is still not appropriate for biopsy application; however, with a few minor changes in the construction of the unit, this no longer will be true.

SUMMARY

To overcome the limitations of sonography and laparoscopy for abdominal diseases, we investigated the use of laparoscopic sonography. The instruments used were the third prototype of the mechanical radial canner, Olympus LPS-UM1/EUM1, and the first prototype of electronic sonolaparoscope of 7.5 MHz made by Olympus Co.

Two hundred eighteen cases were examined with the equipment. The prime importance of the method is its capability to detect and differentiate the occult lesions of the liver, cysts, tumors, various benign focal hyperplasia, and various granulomata. Sonolaparoscopy serves as an excellent modality for visualization of the small mass lesions of the liver as well as provides detailed diagnostic findings that can be used for differential diagnosis of tumors with difficult diagnostic problems.

Acknowledgment

This study was supported in part by a Grant-in-Aid for Cancer Research (60-1) from the Ministry of Health and Welfare, Japan and Grant-in-Aid for Cancer Detection from Keidan-ren.

References

1. Aramaki N, Yoshida K, Yamashiro Y, Namihisa T: Ultrasonic laparoscopy. Scan J Gastroenterol 17 (Suppl 78): 185, 1982.
2. Beck K: Farbatlas der Laparoskopie, 2 Aufl. F. K. Schattauer, Stuttgart, 1980.
3. Boenhof JA, Linhart P, Bettendorf U, Holper H: Liver biopsy guided by laparoscopic sonography. Endoscopy 16: 237–239, 1984.
4. Boenhof JA, Frank K, Loch EG, Linhart P: Laparoscopic sonography. Ann Radiol 28: 16–18, 1985.
5. Frank K, Bliesze H, Boenhof JA, Beck K, Hammes P, Linhart P: Laparoscopic sonography: A new approach to intraabdominal disease. J Clin Ultrasound 13: 60–65, 1985.
6. Fukuda M, Hirata K, Saito K: Studies on intraluminal echography in abdominal diseases: Echolaparoscopy. In Kurjak A (ed): Proceedings of the fourth European Congress on Ultrasonics in Medicine, International Congress Series 547, Excerpta Medica, Amsterdam, 1981, p 109.
7. Fukuda M, Mima S, Nakano Y: Studies on echolaparoscopy. Scan J Gastroenterol 17 (Suppl 78): 186, 1982.
8. Fukuda M, Mima S, Tanabe T, Haniu T, Suzuki Y, Hirata K, Terada S: Endoscopic sonography of the liver, diagnostic application of the echo-laparoscope to localize intrahepatic lesions. Scand J Gastroenterol 19 (Suppl 102): 24–38, 1984.
9. Fukuda M: Use of echoendoscope and echolaparoscope in the diagnosis of intraabdominal cancer. In Kossoff G, Fukuda M (eds): Ultrasonic Differential Diagnosis of Tumors. Igaku-Shoin, New York, 1984, pp 183–199.
10. Itaya H, Fukuda M, Mima S: Studies on early detection of hepatocellular carcinoma. HCC cases detected by ultrasound mass survey with subsequent therapeutic results. In Hepatocellular Carcinoma in Asia, International Center for Medical Research, Kobe University, Kobe, 1984, pp 183–196.
11. Kodama T, Okita K, Oda M: Development and clinical investigation of ultrasonic laparoscopy. Scan J Gastroenterol 17 (Suppl 78): 1, 1982.
12. Saito K, Hirata K, Terada S, Fukuda M, Mima S, Ogura H, Itaya H: Efficient mass survey of liver cell cancer by ultrasound. J Mass Survey Digest Dis 61: 75, 1983.
13. Sheu JC, Sung JL, Chen DS, Yu JY, Wang TH, Su CT, Tsang YM: Ultrasonography of small hepatic tumors using high resolution linear array realtime instrument. Radiology 150: 797–802, 1984.
14. Yamanaka T, Sakai Y, Yoshida Y: Ultrasonic endoscopy for the diagnosis of abdominal lessions 1. Clinical evaluation of an ultrasonic gastroenteroscope with electronic linear scanning system (prototype). Gastroenterol Endosc 24: 607, 1982.

12A

Future Perspectives in Endoscopic Ultrasound

William R. Lees

There has been a great updating in interest in invasive ultrasound scanning in the past few years. There are special ultrasound probes available for scanning within the upper and lower gastrointestinal tracts, from the vagina, the urethra or bladder, and within the abdominal or thoracic cavity during open surgery. Considerable experience has now proved that these techniques provide images of a quality unobtainable by other methods. There is improved spatial and contrast resolution, but this is gained by reducing the field of view.

There is a large number of different design parameters, and many more potential configurations, each of which could prove ideal for a specific clinical application. The development of instruments to study the upper and lower GI tracts and contiguous organs has been the most difficult task for the ultrasound engineers because the instruments must be long and flexible, yet easily manipulated and capable of guidance under direct endoscopic vision. This development is still at an early stage and there remain many technical deficiencies with the present generation of endoprobes which are a compromise between ultrasound and endoscopic technologies.

Most currently available ultrasound endoscopes are large with a long rigid tip that makes endoscopic manipulation difficult; the ultrasound transducer at the end of the instrument is very vulnerable to physical damage or disturbance of its electrical connections. No single design seems suitable for all applications in the GI tract, and future developments will yield a range of instruments rather than an all-purpose device.

Technical development will occur in four areas:

1. The quality of the ultrasound image will improve, and doppler studies will be possible.
2. The endoscopes will become slimmer and less rigid with improved manipulation.
3. The optics will improve.
4. The next generation of instruments will have a biopsy channel, which is currently not available.

ULTRASONOGRAPHIC DEVELOPMENTS

In conventional abdominal ultrasonography, the single crystal transducer has been replaced by multi-element transducers with electronic focusing and beam steering. These new transducers can take advantage of the full power of computer processing to improve resolution and

"

reduce artifacts. However, there are many problems associated with adapting these instruments for intracavity use. It is difficult to construct high-frequency transducer arrays, and even harder to make them small enough to mount on endoscopes. Their resolution is a function of the number of transmitting and receiving elements within the transducer; the most powerful have up to 128 separately wired elements, which results in a bulky cable that cannot be channeled within an endoscope. It will be many years before microelectronics can overcome this particular problem.

Transducers with a limited number of elements have been successfully deployed in the esophagus where they have great advantages in cardiac scanning and in the study of paraesophageal blood flow, such as in varices. The electronic instruments can scan at the high frame rates required to rapidly moving cardiac structures and can now perform two-dimensional doppler blood flow mapping, superimposing the blood-flow pattern on the real-time image by simultaneous color overlay. Such instruments have already been used for diagnosis of varices and for planning and monitoring of injection sclerotherapy (12).

High-frequency single crystal transducers are easy to make, and 10-MHz devices are now in routine use to study the walls of the esophagus, stomach, and duodenum. Frequencies of 15 MHz or higher could result in axial and lateral resolutions of 0.1 and 0.25 mm respectively, but will still have the 2 to 3 cm penetration needed to show the whole gut wall. Very high-frequency transducers could be designed sufficiently small to pass down the biopsy channel of a conventional endoscope. An experimental 17-MHz transducer of this type has been designed by Silverstein. This has fascinating potential not only for study of GI wall lesions but for scanning within the lumen of the biliary tract (10).

ENDOSCOPIC DEVELOPMENTS

The large diameter and long rigid segment of current instruments presents a major handicap. Many esophageal strictures cannot be passed without prior dilation or fear of rupture. In practice, survey of the upper extent of the esophageal tumor and its associated nodal metastases will determine inoperability in more than 95% of cases, whether the stricture has been passed or not, but full staging is not achieved in up to 40% of cases. Experimental esophageal probes without optics do exist. These have external diameters of 8 or 9 mm and can be passed through all but the tightest esophageal strictures.

Removing the optical channel makes the instrument smaller with a more flexible tip. If a forward-facing biopsy channel were provided, the endoscope could be passed over a guidewire as far as the distal duodenum using conventional radiological or endoscopic techniques. Such an instrument would be as manipulable as the conventional fiberoptic endoscope and also would be considerably cheaper than the full combined instrument.

It is legitimate to question the requirement for the combination of flexible endoscopy and ultrasongography for many applications in the GI tract. Study of organs contiguous to the GI tract can be made with the viscus collapsed; navigation and manipulation of the instrument is performed from the ultrasound anatomy alone.

Simultaneous endoscopic and ultrasonographic viewing are mutually incompatable at present but has been performed experimentally and will become a standard feature. The most difficult task with current instruments is passing the pylorus, which cannot be done with ultrasound guidance alone. Even here, a "blind" ultrasound instrument could be passed into the duodenum over a guidewire previously placed by fluoroscopic or conventional endoscopic guidance. It is also debatable whether two degrees of freedom of the tip deflection are required since sufficient steering can be achieved with a single degree of freedom and good torque control.

Suction and insufflation channels are required, as is an additional channel for a standoff balloon to be inflated around the transducer housing. These balloons need to be large enough to obtain 2 to 3 cm of displacement from the gastrointestinal wall. Simplifying the endoscope by removing the fiberoptics would make it easier to manipulate (albeit under fluoroscopic control) as well as make room for an additional biopsy channel.

CLINICAL APPLICATIONS

ESOPHAGUS

Evidence now shows that transesophageal endosonography is the most accurate method of staging esophageal cancer in terms of depth of invasion, length of the invaded segment, and the presence of associated lymphadenopathy (5). The largest series reported so far is that of the Amsterdam group, who have shown an accuracy in determining depth of invasion of better than 75% in a series of more than 70 patients (13). Other large series have shown similar results. Despite promising results obtained by CT scanning in the late 1970s, more recent series have shown that this technique is, in practice, relatively inaccurate and in particular stands very poorly in a direct comparison with EUS (6).

STOMACH

The role of EUS in staging gastric cancer is well established, but provision of a biopsy channel within the instrument is an essential development. This should provide not only for conventional mucosal biopsy forceps, of the type traditionally associated with endoscopy, but also a fine-needle manipulator to drive the needle tip under ultrasound control into the submucosa and muscularis layers, and even into associated lymph nodes and contiguous organs. The sensitivity of ultrasound in detecting celiac axis and perigastric lymph nodes is very high, but the specificity of the technique in discriminating malignant from reactive change is not as good. Although specific signs have been reported for malignant nodes, the accuracy of discrimination is between 75 and 90% (1).

A biopsy channel also allows passage of a miniature doppler ultrasound probe, which can be placed in direct contact with the gastric wall. This is of value in patients with bleeding gastric ulcers, because mapping the blood flow patterns around the ulcer crater allows determination of the most appropriate site for the application of laser, heater probes, or sclerosants (2). Preliminary experiments with endosonographic monitoring of laser therapy of esophageal and gastric cancer show that the two techniques are complementary. Thus, EUS control becomes more important with subsequent treatments when the fibrosis induced by laser makes navigation of the beam hazardous (4).

DUODENAL LOOP

The long rigid tip of the conventional instrument makes passage through the pylorus and in the second part of the duodenum extremely difficult. In our fifth year of experience with upper GI endosonography, we still have a failure rate of approximately 10% in reaching the region of the ampulla. In a small percentage of patients, such discomfort is experienced in this process that even though the duodenum can be intubated (a poor quality study is obtained). Improvements in endoscope design will minimize this problem but provision of a forward-emerging guidewire would be an enormous advantage.

GALLBLADDER AND PORTA HEPATIS

The region of the liver hilum is difficult to visualize reliably with radially-scanning ultrasound endoscopes, but this is an important area to assess in all patients with biliary or pancreatic disease. The problem is that the axis of the pylorus and duodenal cap points toward the porta hepatis, and the radial instrument scans at 90% to this plane. A forward view would open up new areas of biliary tract scanning.

PANCREAS

After placing the ultrasound tip in the second part of the duodenum distal to the ampulla of Vater, it is possible to withdraw the endoscope slowly along the duodenum, through the pylorus and along the curve of the stomach, and see the entire pancreas in over 80% of patients. The anatomy of the pancreatic duct can be mapped by tracking the endoscope with lateral tip deflection, and the main pancreatic duct and its major branches are clearly seen in most normal subjects.

The high soft-tissue contrast resolution of the instrument can discriminate the ventral from dorsal anlages of the pancreas, which have a different histological structure. The dorsal pancreas appears more echogenic than the ventral and the division between the two is clearly seen. This is important because most of the false-positive diagnoses of tumors of the head of the pancreas on CT scanning are caused by variations in size of the ventral segments. Current indications for EUS of the pancreas are:

1. Evaluation of the pancreatic mass where discrimination between chronic pancreatitis and cancer is not possible by CT or conventional ultrasound.
2. Staging of small pancreatic neoplasms before surgery.
3. Detection of islet cell tumors.
4. Evaluation of localized areas of abnormality of the main pancreatic duct as shown by pancreatography that are not resolved by conventional invasive imaging.
5. Discrimination of the normal pancreas from early chronic pancreatitis in patients with pain of probable pancreatic origin.
6. Mapping the distribution of changes in early chronic pancreatitis with particular reference to the relative damage to the duct and parenchyma.

For most of these indications, EUS is the technique of choice; for the others, it is the final technique performed before surgery or biopsy. In our practice, approximately 10% of patients with pancreatic pathology receive EUS. It has been firmly established as the most specific diagnostic modality. This technique for pancreatic endosonography is effective and is unlikely to be improved further except by the addition of the guided-needle biopsy facility (7).

LOWER GASTROINTESTINAL TRACT

"Blind" rigid ultrasound endoscopes have been used very effectively for staging rectal cancer and for detecting recurrence. This is shown to be much more sensitive than CT scanning or digital examination (3, 9). The depth of penetration through the various layers of the rectal wall is clearly demonstrated, as is invasion of the serosa and perirectal fat. Advanced rectal cancer is not seen as well as with CT or MRI because the full extent of invasion of the pelvic side walls and presacral fossa cannot be seen so clearly and the superior extent of invasion is very difficult to demonstrate with the conventional rigid instruments. Perirectal nodal involvement is very clearly seen, but reactive hyperplasia in pelvic nodes is common. The ability of EUS to discriminate inflammatory from malignant involvement is no better than 75%.

It is difficult to use the same instruments for rectal and colonic endosonography as for the upper GI tract, but there is no doubt that an instrument with the range and maneuverability of a colonoscope would greatly enhance the power of this technique. Endosonography in this area is unlikely to displace CT or MRI, which will remain necessary for their exquisite ability to demonstrate pelvic side-wall involvement and more distant nodal metastases. However, a combination of EUS and CT or MRI is much more accurate than any one technique alone (8).

An ultrasonic colonoscope will have important applications in inflammatory bowel disease.

ECONOMICS OF ENDOSONOGRAPHY

Rigid transrectal and transvaginal endosonography are now widely used and are well established in ultrasound imaging. Progress in development has been slow, and it is now almost 20 years since Watanabe first described the initial transrectal experience with the Aloka Chair (14). The recent popularity of this technique has resulted largely from economic as well as scientific factors. Mechanical and electronic transrectal and transvaginal probes are now cheap, readily available from most manufacturers, and can be interfaced to existing conventional ultrasound equipment. In many hospitals, machines are dedicated solely to transrectal or transvaginal endosonography, but nearly all these machines are in the bottom third of the price range for ultrasound apparatus.

World-wide acceptance of the combined fiberoptic and ultrasound endoscope has been much slower despite firm scientific evidence as to its effectiveness. Its limitation has been a combination of high price (in the top third of the ultrasound price range) and logistic difficulties.

If upper GI endosonography is to become a routine clinical tool, it must become easier to use and be capable of interfacing with existing ultrasound equipment. It is easy to envision every ultrasound department having at least one ultrasound machine that can be used in the upper GI tract, rectum, or in the operating theater with intraoperative probes. Such a machine should not be priced above the middle third of the ultrasound price range and the probes should be rugged and cheap. Eventually it is likely that most routine upper GI endoscopic ultrasound will be performed with instruments without associated fiberoptics, and the more expensive combined instruments will be confined to a few academic centers.

Endosonography is still at a very early stage of development and lags behind the state of the art in extracorporeal ultrasound. Further development will depend as much on commercial as scientific interest.

ACCEPTANCE OF ENDOSONOGRAPHY BY GASTROENTEROLOGISTS

Before there is widespread use of endosonography in the upper and lower GI tracts, its proponents must establish that the technique is safe and well tolerated, that information is obtained that cannot be gained by noninvasive methods, and that this information will benefit patient management.

The last few years have seen the painstaking acquisition of real data and those working in the field believe its value is established in staging cancer of the esophagus, stomach, and rectum and in postoperative follow-up. Studies of the pancreas and liver are less obviously beneficial, except in the context of highly specialized referral centers. Paradoxically, the greatest threat of future prospects of endosonography will come from improvement in conventional ultrasound equipment rather than from CT or MRI.

References

1. Aibe T, Ito T, Yoshida T, Noguchi T, Ohtani T, Fuji T, Takemoto T: Endoscopic ultrasonography of lymph nodes surrounding the upper GI tract. Scand J Gastroenterol 21 (Suppl 123): 164–170, 1986.
2. Beckley D: Personal communication.
3. Beynon J, Foy DM, Roe AM, Temple LN, Mortensen NJ: Endoluminal ultrasound in the assessment of local invasion in rectal carcinoma. Br J Surg 6: 474–477, 1986.
4. Bown SG: Endoscopic laser therapy for esophageal cancer. Endoscopy 18 (Suppl 3): 26–31, 1986.
5. Dancygier H, Classen M: How can we diagnose the depth of cancer invasion in the esophagus? Endoscopy 18 (Suppl 3): 19–21, 1986.
6. Lea JW, Prager RL, Bender Jr HW: The questionable role of computed tomography in preoperative staging of esophageal cancer. Ann Thorac Surg 38: 479, 1984.
7. Lees WR: Endoscopic ultrasonography of chronic pancreatitis and pancreatic pseudocysts. Scand J Gastroenterol 21 (Suppl 123): 123–129, 1986.
8. Meyer JE, Dosoretz DE, Gunderson LL, Stark P, Kopans DB: CT evaluation of locally advanced carcinoma of the distal colon and rectum. J Compt Assist Tomogr 7: 265–267, 1983.
9. Rifkin MD, McGlynn ET, Marks G: Endorectal sonographic prospective staging of rectal cancer. Scand J Gastroenterol 21 (Suppl 123): 99–103, 1986.
10. Silverstein F, Kimmey M, Martin R, Haggitt R, Mack A, Moss A, Franklin D: Ultrasound and intestinal wall: Experimental methods. Scand J Gastroenterol 21 (Suppl 123): 34–40, 1986
11. Strohm WD, Classen M: Benign lesions of the upper GI tract by means of endoscopic ultrasonography. Scand J Gastroenterol 21 (Suppl 123): 41–46, 1986.
12. Sukigara et al.: Colour flow mapping of esophagogastric varices and vessels in and around the liver with real-time two dimensional doppler echography. Clin Radiol (in press)
13. Tio TL, Den Hartog Jager FCA, Tytgat GNJ: The role of endoscopic ultrasonography in assessing local resectability of esophagogastric malignancies. Accuracy, pitfalls and predictability. Scand J Gastroenterol 21 (Suppl 123): 78–86, 1986.
14. Watanabe H, Saitoh M, Mishina T, Igari D, Tanahashi Y, Harada K, Hisamichi S: Mass screening program for prostatic diseases with transrectal ultrasonotomography. J Urol 117: 746–748, 1977.

12B

Perspectives of Endoscopic Ultrasonography:
A Review from a Medical Engineer's Viewpoint

Kazuo Baba

Almost eight years have passed since the first prototype of ultrasound endoscope was produced. The equipment that we developed was really one of the so-called "barrack" models and had a number of defects to be worked out. The observed images were barely discernible on a small CRT of the unit, and it was frequently necessary to use many packs of expensive Polaroid film. Consequently, we had to spend a fairly long time fixing any defects that occurred in the instruments during their experimental use on clinical cases. However, it is our pleasure to see that the very feeble test model has recently gained a good reputation among clinicians, who are critical in using any kind of instrument in the clinical practice of gastroenterology, especially in the field of gastrointestinal endoscopy.

The rigid ultrasonic scanner had been used in the rectal lumen without endoscopic devices, but no apparatus equipped with the endoscope was available until recently. This innovation occurred at two places, in Nagoya, Japan, by Hisanaga and co-workers, and in Palo Alto, California, by P.S. Green of SRI. Hisanaga first attempted to record ultrasonic tomograms from the esophageal lumen using an intraesophageal transducer without an endoscopic outfit, whereas Green tried to scan the pancreas with a linear-array probe attached to the tip of the gastrofiberscope. Like other innovative discoveries in other scientific fields, those researches were carried out and reported independently, the former in the field of cardiology and the latter in collaboration with Mayo staff in the field of radiology. Both papers were reported between 1978 and 1980. To my knowledge, the intraesophageal scanning by hand-made equipment seemed to be awful and intolerable for routine clinical use. I never imagined even to have got involved in manufacturing the prototype equipment.

The ultrasound endoscope has established a firm stand in the clinical practice of gastroenterology. From a medical engineer's viewpoint, however, it is still far from complete, and further innovation is necessary to finish this hot-from-the-oven instrument. Fortunately, a number of troublesome aspects should be worked out in the near future, and this will surely aid the clinicians who are struggling to yield original inspiring works from this still immature piece of equipment.

What troublesome aspects must be improved? It is of primary importance to increase the functional capability of the unit as an endoscope, and to improve the quality of the ultrasonograms that are obtained through such means as switching the suitable transducer frequencies to optimize the image. Other improvements concern the color-mapping rendition by the additive use of Doppler flowmetry and the production of an additive model with ultrasound videoendoscope by the use of an advanced CCD plate. Some of these problems are in the process of development and some will probably be completed in the near future. Especially

138

promising is the combination of the latter two concerns; the image recording through the CCD tip will open up a new area of image processing to be used in more detailed diagnostic means, whereas its combination with Doppler signal processing, especially geared to the low speed flow, will eventually provide potent diagnostic data in cases of malignant neoplasms. The more detailed visualization of the layering structure of the gastrointestinal tract wall by 20 MHz or more frequencies will give a far more accurate determination than before of the extent of cancer infiltration in vivo.   The application of ultrasonic pulse compression will have ample use in the diagnosis of pancreatic carcinoma, whose diagnosis is often troubled by insufficient visualization due to the present stage of equipment development.

Other desired developments, such as the use of ultrasonic tissue characterization, will increase insight to the nature of the tissue under investigation, and direct biopsy by means of ultrasonic guidance is indeed within the scope of the method.   Furthermore, a three-dimensional rendition using sequential serial scannings should be possible with the concommitant use of powerful computer softwares.

Overall, the most urgent task of the engineer is the continuous challenge of improving miniaturization and dependability of the unit itself.   But the largest problem is the vulnerability of the methodology.   The present endoscopic ultrasound equipment is mainly geared to investigating the upper gastrointestinal tract of abdominal cavities.   If it were practicable to use in another type of intraluminal scanning, it will be a great help in routine clinical settings, such as in gynecological, coloproctological, or endobronchial scanning.   Also, its application to cardiovascular diseases is a largely unexplored area, and sector scanning through the esophageal wall together with color flow mapping already suggests its immense use in clinical practice.

The selection of scanning modes, either the mechanical or electronic array system, is still under active debate.   At present, the mechanical scanning mode is far superior in terms of easy manipulation, insertion and ease of image recognition.   However, the future points to the electronic array system because it has no mechanical problems and is maintenance-free.

It is indeed a medical engineer's dream to make a single piece of equipment that incorporates a very small transducer as a scanner and has the endoscope's superior capability.   The ultrasound tip is so small that the endoscopist does not have to insert a bulky ultrasound endoscope, and yet the instrument can be switched to ultrasound endoscope within a second or high quality endoscopic images together with ultrasound images can be seen in parallel on the screen.

We sincerely hope that these developments will be slated for use within a very short time, and endoscopists will no longer be troubled with other types of intricate, expensive, and time-consuming examinations, which are not only troublesome to the physicians but to the patient as well.

13

Anatomical Aspects of Endoscopic Ultrasonography

Kenjiro Yasuda, Keisuke Kiyota, Hidekazu Mukai, Eisai Cho

The endoscopic ultrasonography (EUS) images are obtained by endoscopes that are attached to the ultrasonic transducer at the tip. Sometimes these images are difficult to understand because they are observed from the intraluminal position.

The ultrasonic endoscope has a radial ultrasonic transducer to obtain the 360 degree image around the gastrointestinal canal. Two types of scanning methods are available for clinical use. One is the water-filling method for observing the gastrointestinal wall. The other is the balloon contact method for observing the esophagus and extra canal organs, such as the pancreato-biliary system, mediastinum and perirectal organs.

In these scanning, it is most important to place some sonolucent materials such as water between the lesion and the transducer. So the combined method of water-filling and balloon contact is usually available for all diseases examined by EUS.

In this chapter, we describe the normal and pathological images of EUS and their scanning positions for ease in understanding EUS images.

EUS IMAGES OF NORMAL AND PATHOLOGICAL FINDINGS OF THE GI TRACT

Digestive tract diseases are examined based on the analysis of the layered structure observed by EUS. The lesions in the esophagus, stomach, duodenum, and rectosigmoidal colon can be examined by this method. All the lesions of these digestive canals are observed ultrasonographically through the water, with or without the balloon attached around the ultrasonic transducer.

ESOPHAGEAL WALL AND INTRATHORACIC ORGANS

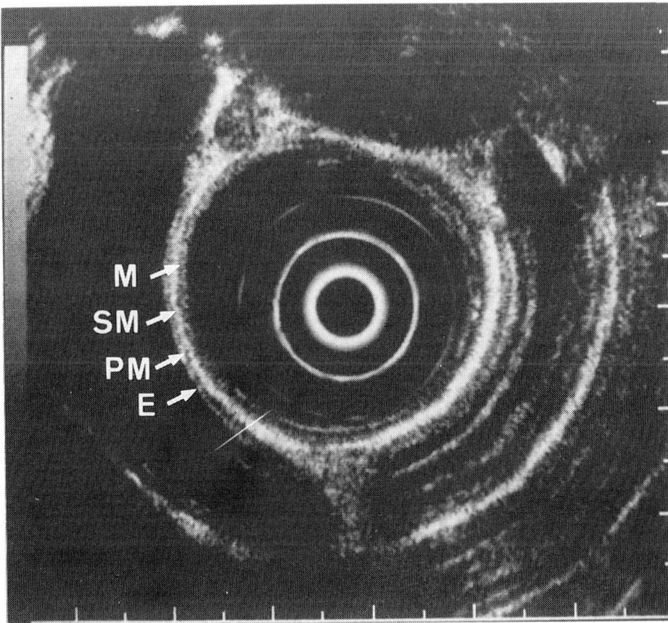

Fig. 13-1. Esophageal wall observed by the water-filling method, showing the five-layered structure. M, mucosa; SM, submucosa; MP, muscularis propria; E, extra canal layer.

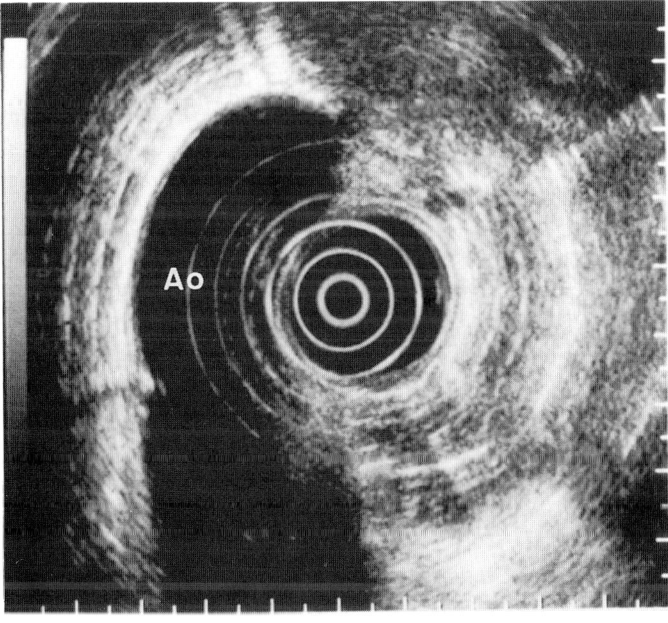

Fig. 13-2A (Legend on page 142)

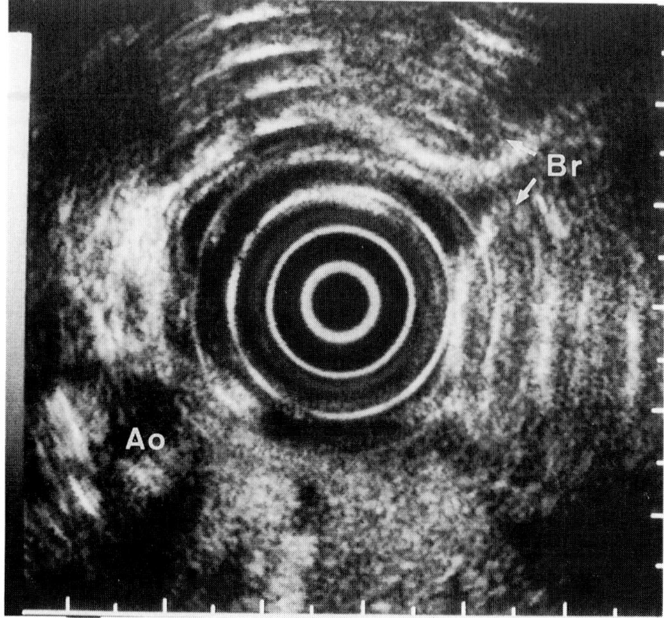

Fig. 13-2B

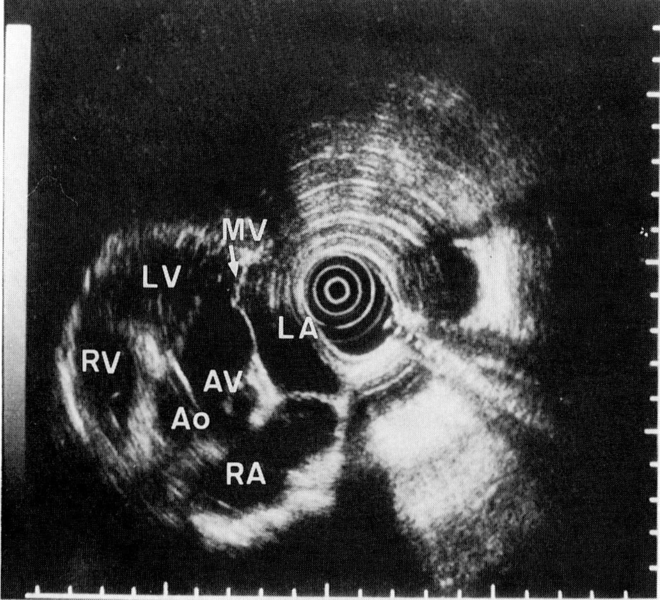

Fig. 13-2C

Fig. 13-2. Intrathoracic findings through the esophageal wall observed by EUS. **A.** EUS picture from the upper esophagus. Aortic arch (Ao) is observed. **B.** EUS picture from the middle portion of the esophagus; bilateral bronchus (Br) are observed showing acoustic shadows at the opposite side descending aorta (Ao). **C.** From the lower portion of the esophagus, the heart is observed as a cross section (LA, left atrium; LV, left ventricle; RA, right atrium; RV, right ventricle; Ao, aorta; MV, mitral valve; AV, aortic valve).

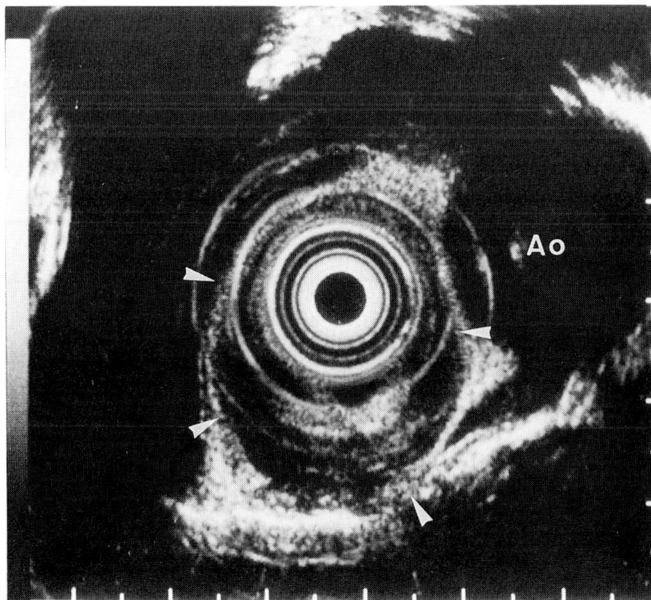

Fig. 13-3. EUS image of advanced carcinoma of the esophagus. The echogram of the tumor mass (arrows) shows the destruction of the layered structure of the esophageal wall.

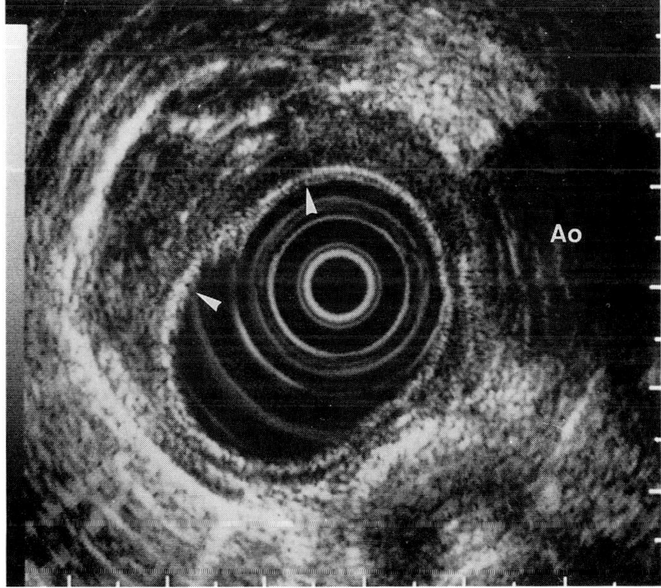

Fig. 13-4. EUS image of submucosal tumor of the middle esophagus (arrows) locating in the muscularis propria. The tumor showing the echogenic spots was histologically revealed to be a leiomyoma.

NORMAL GASTRIC WALL AND PATHOLOGICAL CHANGE OF THE GASTRIC WALL OBSERVED BY ENDOSCOPIC ULTRASONOGRAPHY

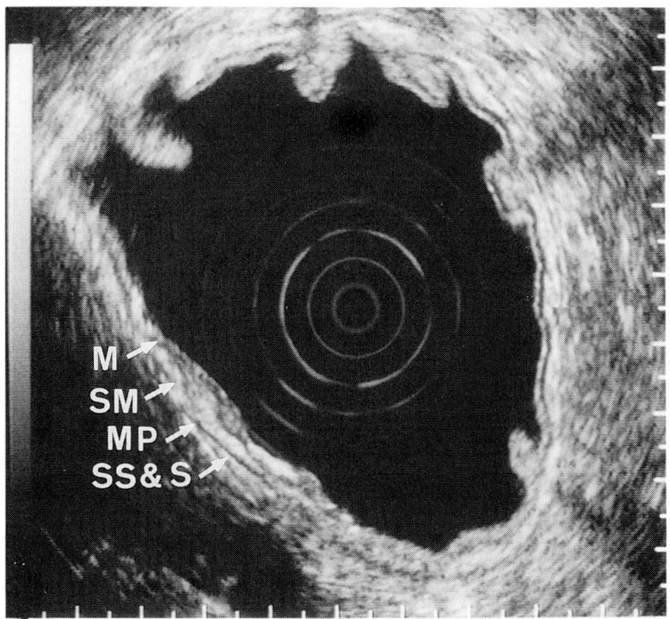

Fig. 13-5A   (Legend on page 145)

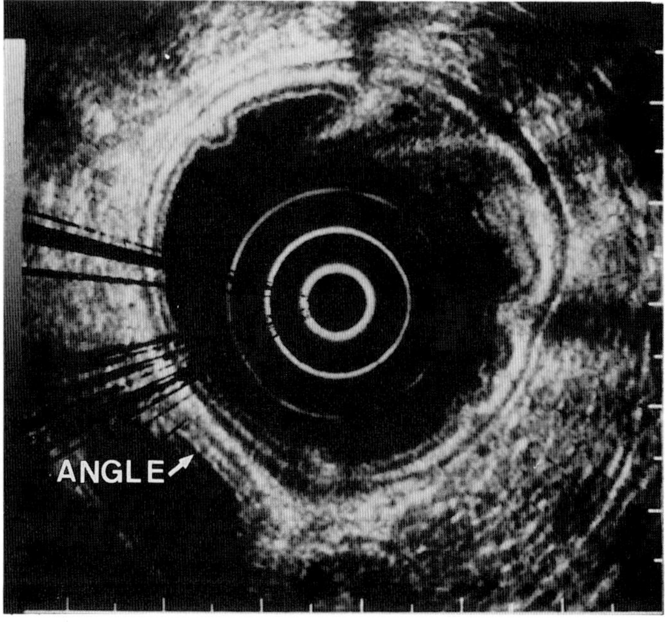

Fig. 13-5B   (Legend on page 145)

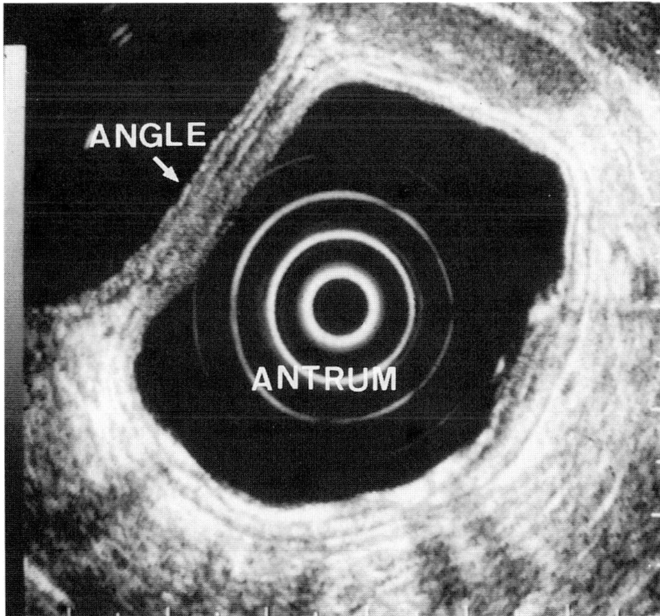

Fig. 13-5C

Fig. 13-5. EUS images of the normal gastric wall. **A.** The upper body of the stomach showing the five-layered structure (M, mucosa; SM, submucosa; MP, muscularis propria; SS, S, subserosa, serosa). **B.** The angle of the stomach showing the double five-layered structure. **C.** The antrum of the stomach showing the same layered structure.

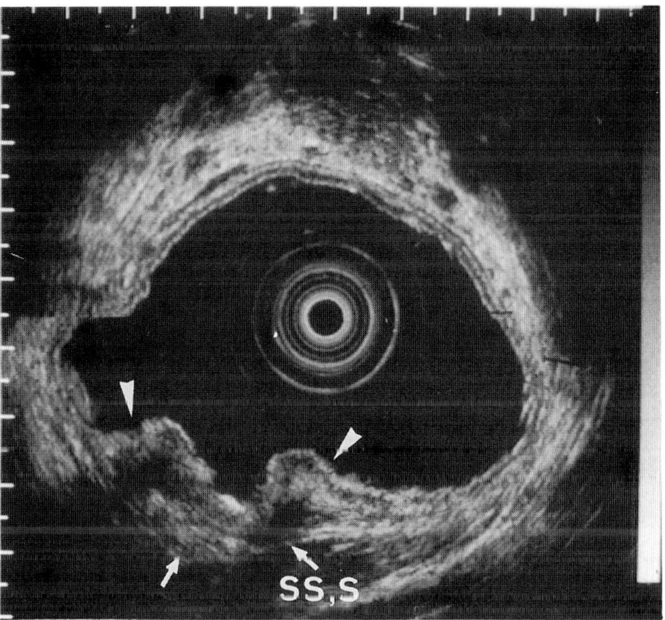

Fig. 13-6A (Legend on page 146)

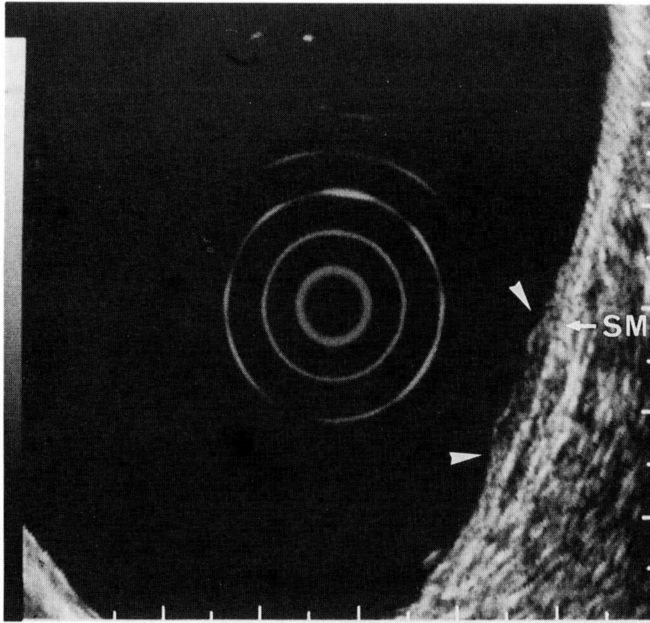

Fig. 13-6B

Fig. 13-6.   EUS images of carcinoma of the stomach.   **A.** Advanced carcinoma Borrmann type III; the tumor mass (arrow heads) destructing and penetrating the gastric wall into the serosal layer (arrows). **B.** Early carcinoma limited to the mucosa (arrow heads; Type IIc) showing the mucosal change with no abnormality of the submucosal layer.

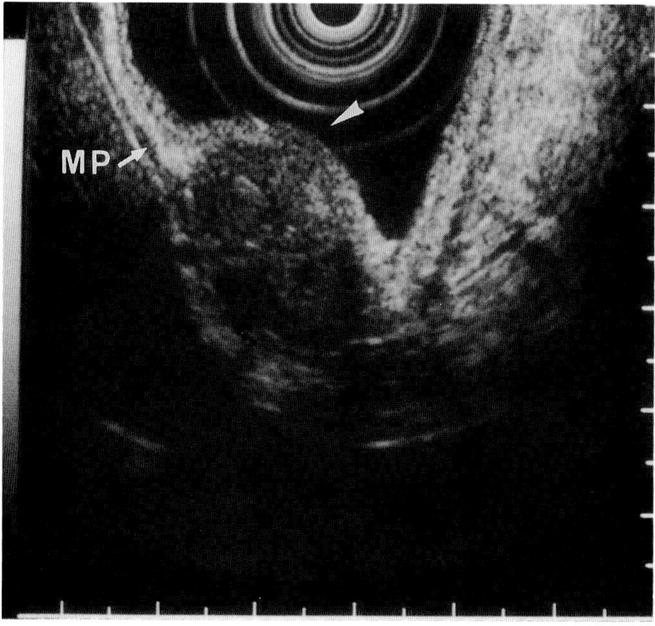

Fig. 13-7A   (Legend on page 147)

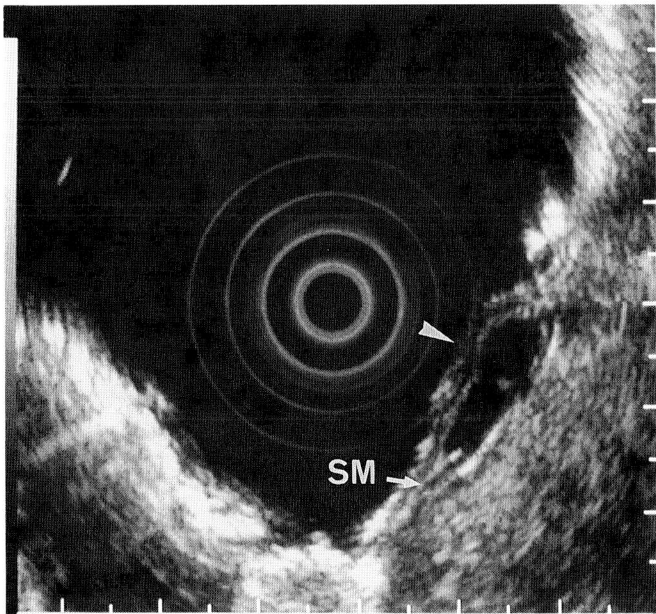

Fig. 13-7B

Fig. 13-7. EUS images of a submucosal tumor (SMT) of the stomach. **A.** Leiomyoma; a round hypo-echoic tumor (arrow) shows the irregular inner echogram and the continuity with the fourth hypoechoic proper muscle layer (MP). **B.** Cyst; a round, echo-free lesion (arrow) is observed in the third hyperechoic submucosal layer (SM).

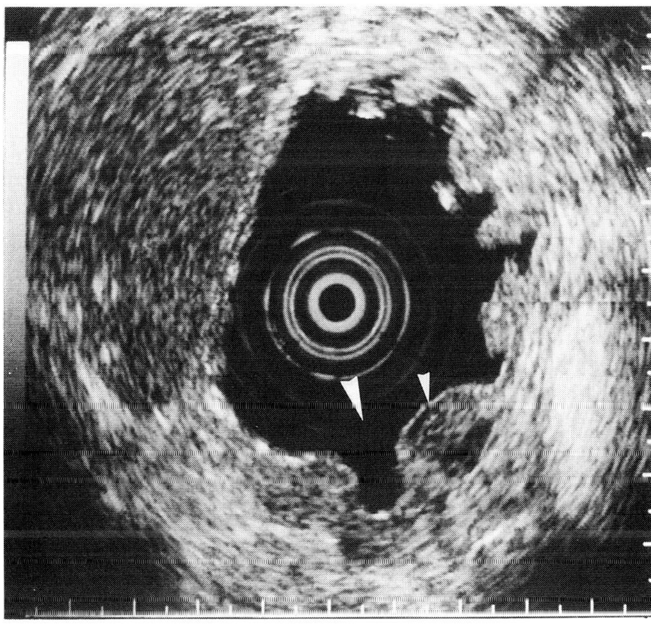

Fig. 13-8A (Legend on page 148)

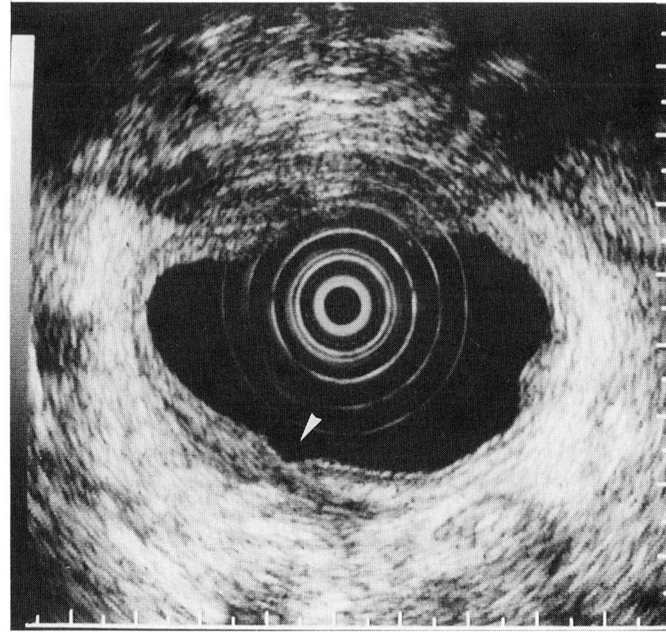

Fig. 13-8B

Fig. 13-8.   EUS images of a peptic ulcer of the stomach.   **A.** An active ulcer shows the defect of the ulcer (large arrow) and the swelling of the surrounding wall (small arrow).   **B.** The scar of a peptic ulcer shows the centrization of the layers to the point of the ulcer scar (arrow).

ENDOSCOPIC ULTRASONOGRAPHIC IMAGES OF THE DUODENAL WALL

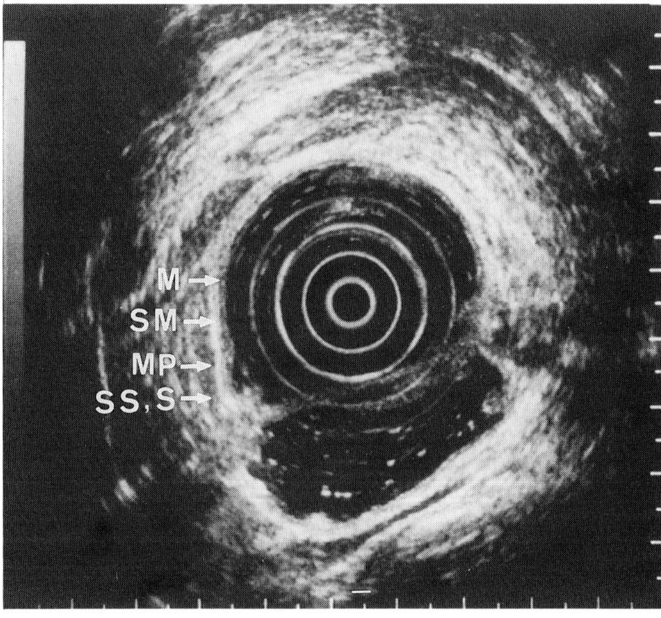

Fig. 13-9A   (Legend on page 149)

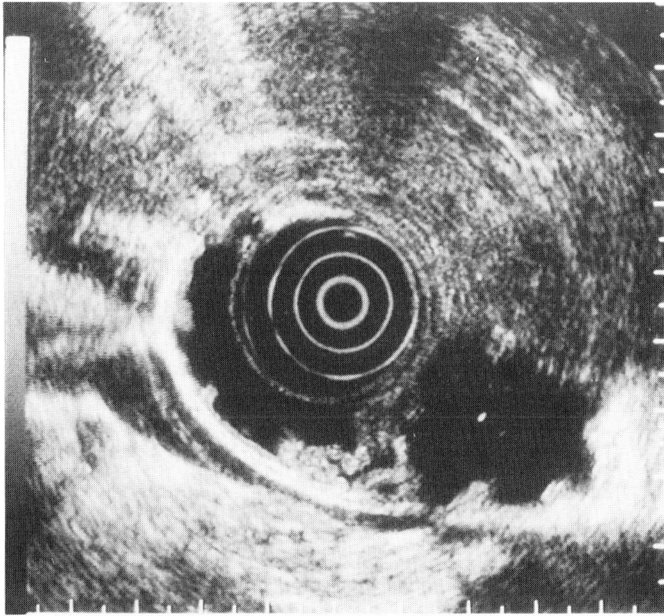

Fig. 13-9B

Fig. 13-9. Normal EUS images of the duodenal wall. **A.** Duodenal wall observed by the water-filling method showing the five-layered structure. **B.** Duodenal second portion observed by the water-filling method.

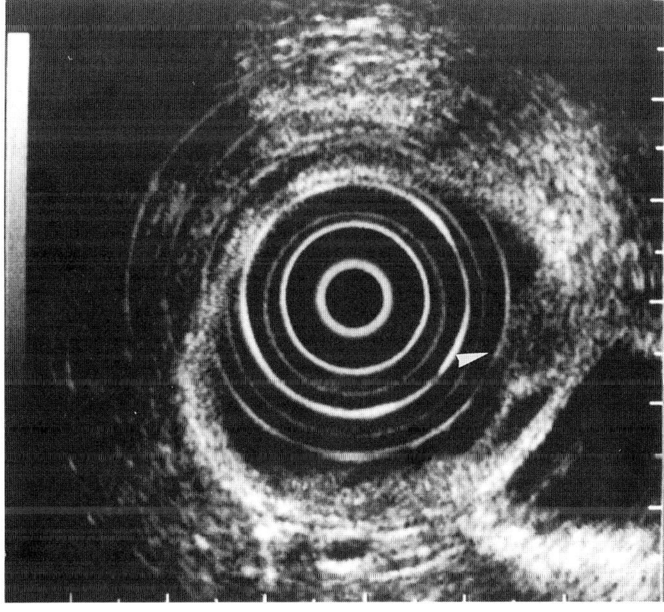

Fig. 13 10. EUS image of the bulnerioma of the duodenum showing a hyperechoic solid tumor (arrow).

NORMAL AND PATHOLOGICAL FINDINGS OF THE RECTOSIGMOID COLON AND PERIRECTAL ORGANS

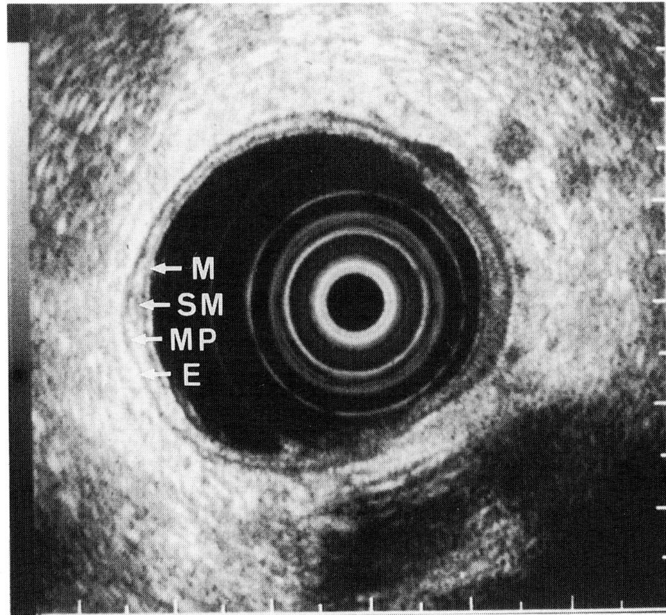

Fig. 13-11A

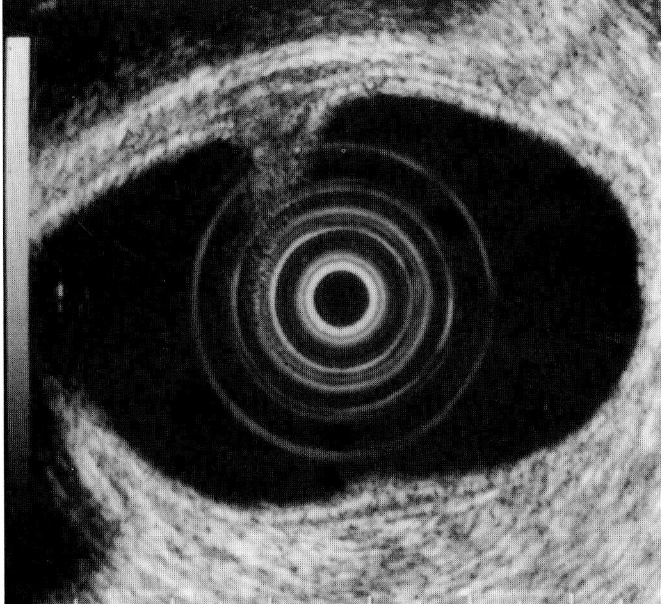

Fig. 13-11B

Fig. 13-11. Normal EUS images of the rectosigmoid colon. **A.** The rectal wall observed by the water-filling method showing the five-layered structure. The fifth layer is the border line with the intrapelvic organs. **B.** The sigmoid colon wall showing the five-layered structure, same as that of the gastric wall.

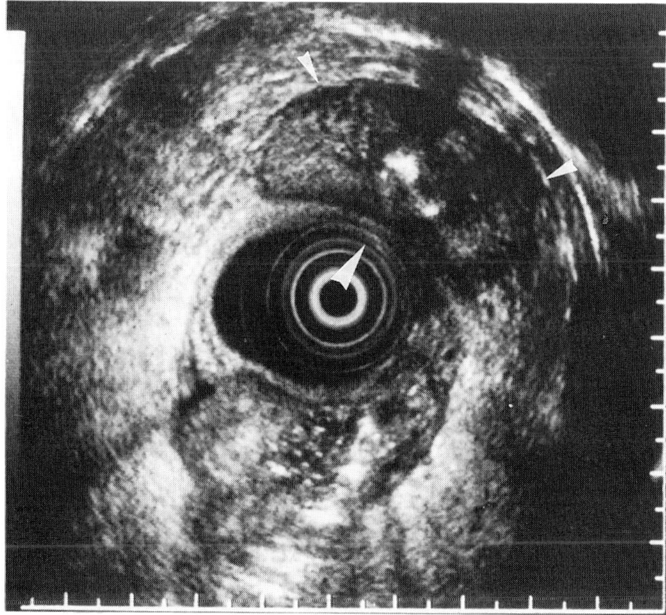

Fig. 13-12A

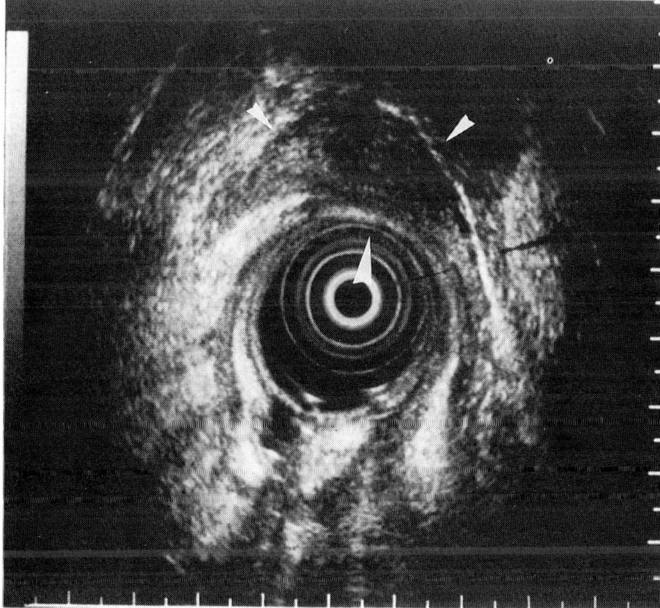

Fig. 13-12B

Fig. 13-12. EUS images of the extrarectal organs. **A.** The prostata (arrows) through the rectal wall. **B.** The uterus (arrows) through the rectal wall.

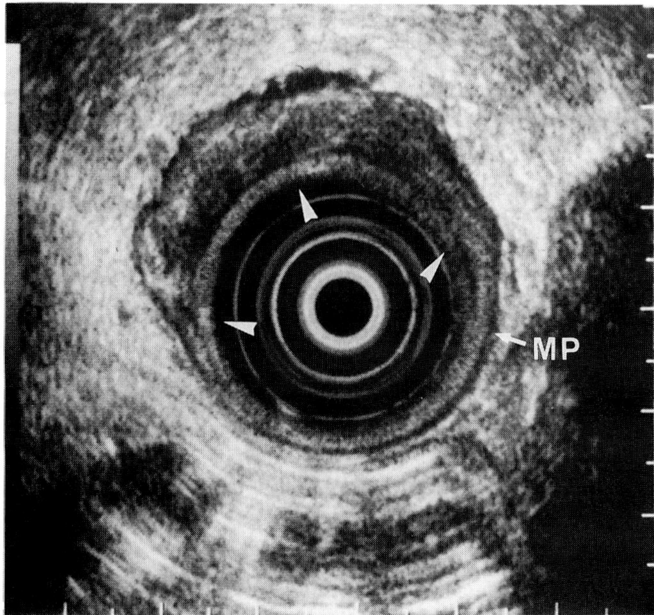

Fig. 13-13A

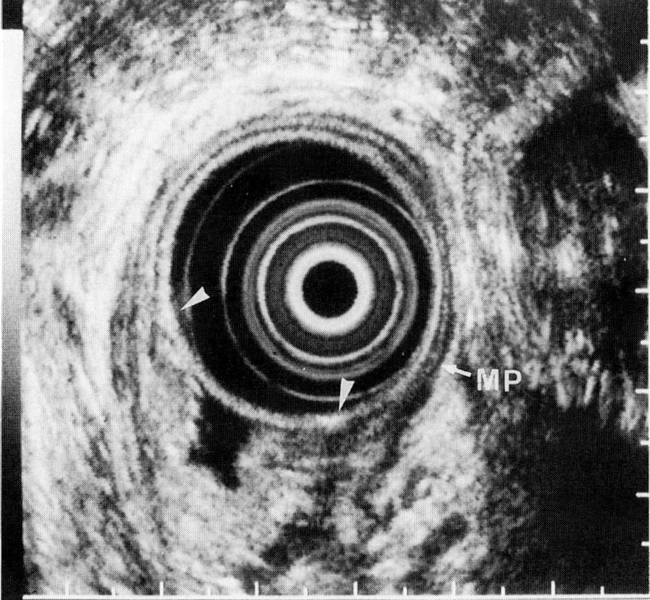

Fig. 13-13B

Fig. 13-13. EUS images of rectosigmoidal carcinoma. **A.** Rectal carcinoma, showing the tumor mass (arrows) destructing the layered structure of the wall. **B.** Sigmoid colon carcinoma (arrows) invading into the extraserosal area, showing the destruction of the layered structure completely.

ENDOSCOPIC ULTRASONOGRAPHIC IMAGES OF NORMAL AND PATHOLOGICAL FINDINGS OF THE HEPATO-PANCREATO-BILIARY SYSTEM

The hepato-pancreato-biliary system is observed through the duodenal and gastric wall by EUS. The pancreas, which was difficult to observe by conventional ultrasonographic tomography (UST), was the most important target organ for EUS from the beginning of the development of this method. On the other hand, the ultrasonographic observations of the liver and gallbladder were sufficient by UST. EUS study for these organs is useful for a further and precise examination technique.

ENDOSCOPIC ULTRASONOGRAPHIC IMAGES OF THE LIVER

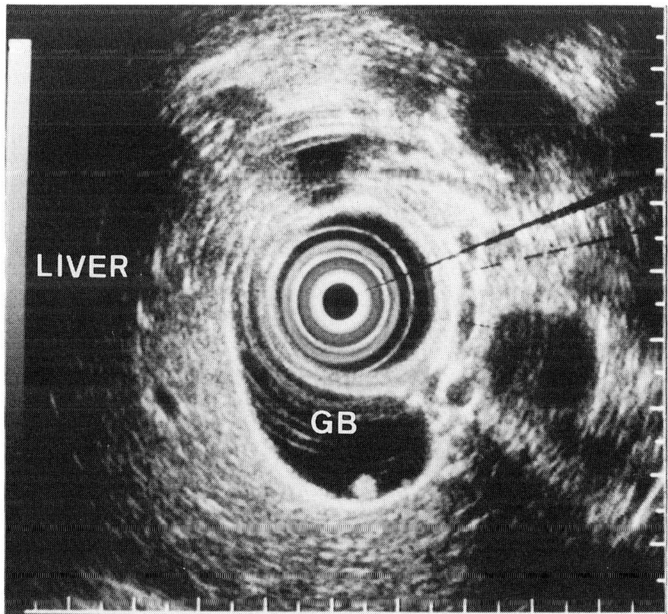

Fig. 13-14A

Fig. 13-14. Normal images of the liver. **A.** The right lobe of the liver through the duodenal wall (GB, gallbaldder). **B.** The left lobe of the liver though the gastric wall (Sp, spleen).

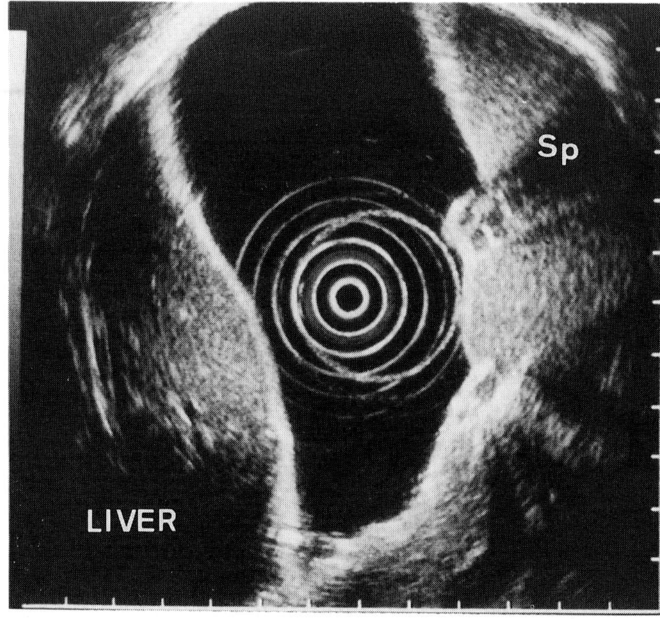

Fig. 13-14B   (Lengend on page 153)

NORMAL AND PATHOLOGICAL ENDSCOPIC ULTRASONOGRAPHIC IMAGES OF THE PANCREAS

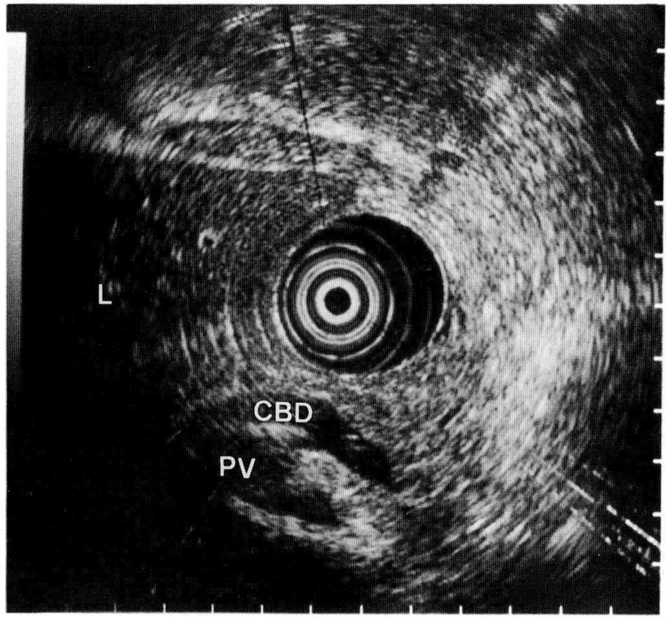

Fig. 13-15A   (Lengend on page 155)

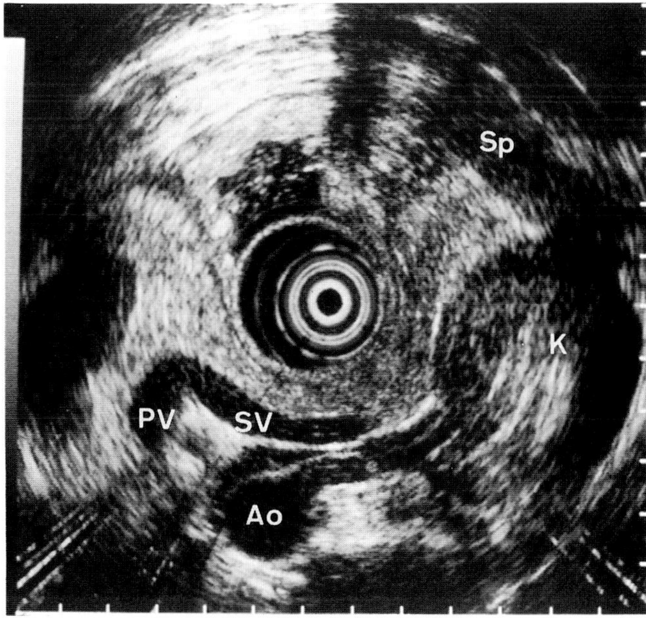

Fig. 13-15B

Fig. 13-15. Normal images of the pancreas. **A.** The head of the pancreas through the duodenal second portion (L, liver; CBD, common bile duct; PV, portal vein). **B.** The body and tail of the pancreas through the gastric wall (SV, splenic vein; K, kidney).

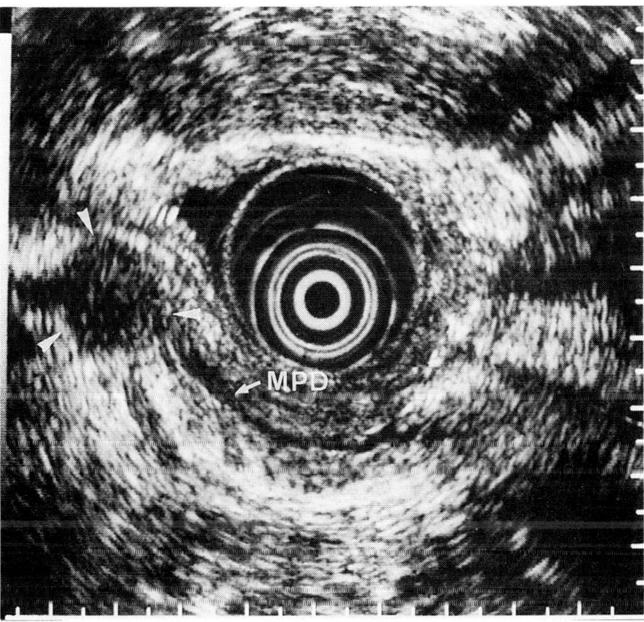

Fig. 13-16A (Lengend on page 156)

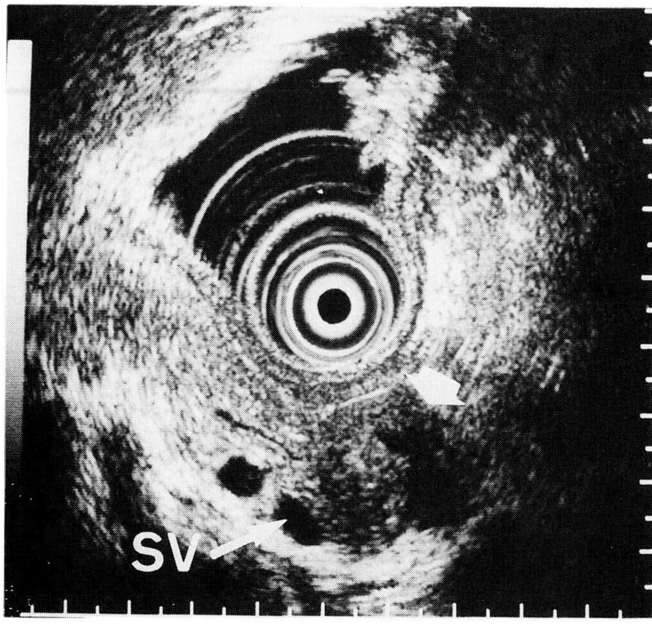

Fig. 13-16B

Fig. 13-16.   EUS images of carcinoma of the pancreas.   **A.** A case of pancreas head carcinoma showing a hypoechoic tumor mass (arrows) at the head of the pancreas with a dilated main pancreatic duct (MPD).   **B.** A case of pancreas tail carcinoma showing a hypoechoic tumor mass with a cystic change at the tail of the pancreas (arrow).

ENDOSCOPIC ULTRASONOGRAPHIC IMAGES OF THE COMMON BILE DUCT AND GALLBLADDER

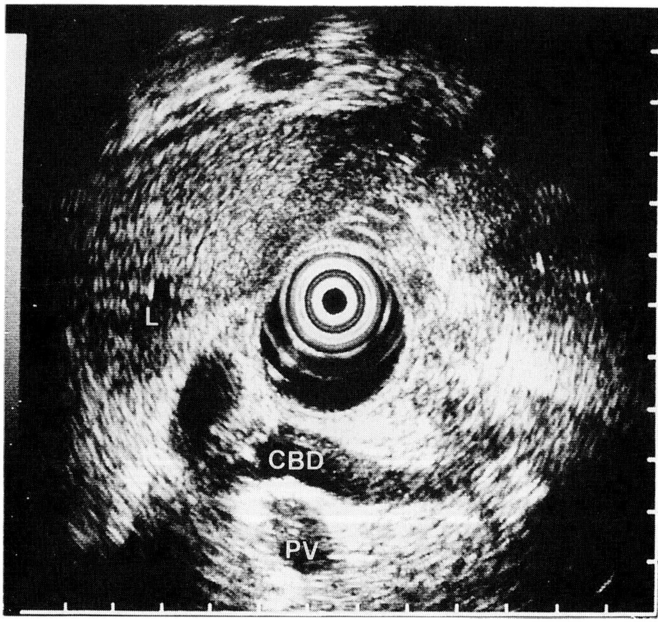

Fig. 13-17A   (Lengend on page 157)

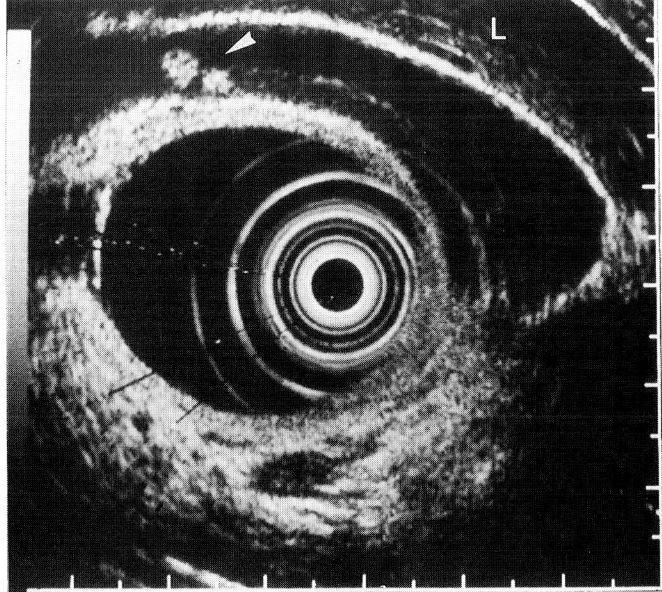

Fig. 13-17B

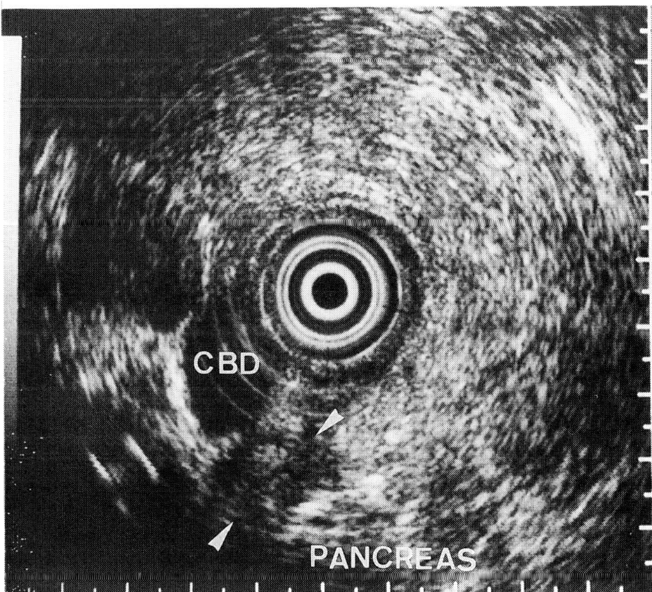

Fig. 13-17C

Fig. 13-17. Normal and pathological images of the biliary tract. **A.** Normal image of the common bile duct (CBD) with that of liver and portal vein through the duodenal second portion. **B.** Normal image of the gall-bladder (GB) demonstrated as a layered structure through the duodenal bulb. The arrow shows cholesterol polyps observed as hyperechoic spots. **C.** A case of choledochal carcinoma showing a hypoechoic tumor at the lower portion of the CBD (arrows).

ENDOSCOPIC ULTRASONOGRAPHIC IMAGES OF THE PAPILLA OF VATER

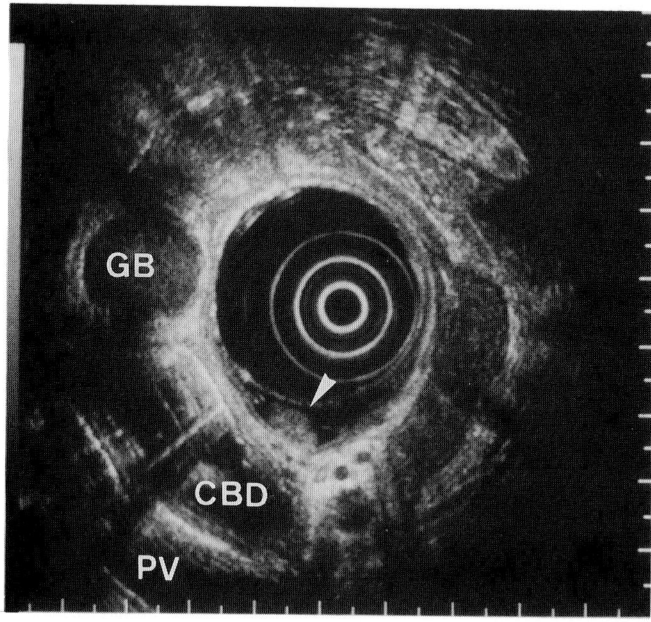

Fig. 13-18A

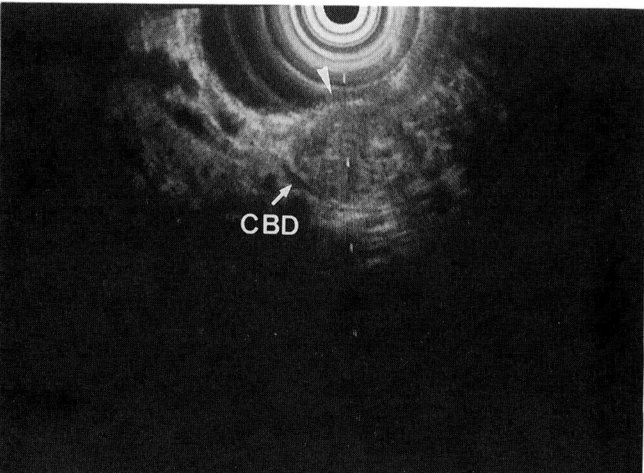

Fig. 13-18B

Fig. 13-18. Normal and pathological images of the papilla of Vater. **A.** Normal image of the papilla of Vater (arrow) showing a layered structure with the common bile duct (CBD), gallbladder (GB), and the portal vein (PV). **B.** A case of the duodenal papilla showing the hypoechoic tumor mass (arrow) destructing the layered structure of the papilla of Vater.

Index

A

Accuracy rate for cancer invasion   64
Acute gastric mucosal lesion   51, 52
Adenomyomatosis of gallbladder   88, 94, 98
AGML   *see* Acute gastric mucosal lesion
Anatomical aspects of digestive organ   5, 140–158

B

Benign gastrointestinal disease   44–55
Bile duct cancer   98, 115
Biliary tract, diseases of   96–101
   normal   97, 157
Bulnerioma of duodenum   149

C

Cancer
   depth of invasion   66
   of bile duct   98, 115
   of colon   68
   of esophagus   60, 61, 106–109
   of gallbladder   95, 117
   of liver   125–127
   of pancreas   72–78, 112
   of papilla of Vater   67, 101
   of stomach   60–67
Cholangiocellular carcinoma   126
Cholecystitis   88
Choledochal stone   98
Cholesterol polyp   90, 98
Chronic pancreatitis   76, 79 86
Colon cancer   68
Colon polyp   54

Colon wall, normal   39, 59, 150
Common bile duct, malignancy in   115
Criteria for depth of cancer invasion   66
Cronkhite-Canada syndrome   53

D

Diagnostic efficiency in pancreatic cancer   77
Dilatation of pancreatic duct   83
Duodenal cancer   67
Duodenal wall, normal   14, 39, 59, 148, 149

E

Echographic pattern of GI wall   38–40, 45
Electronic scanning   18, 19
Endoscopic ultrasonography
   examination technique   3–15
   future perspectives   16, 33, 132, 138
   instrument   2, 29–32
Esophageal cancer   60, 61, 106–109, 143
Esophageal wall, normal   6–8, 38, 57, 58, 141, 142
EUS   *see* Endoscopic ultrasonography
External compression   46

F

Focal nodular hyperplasia   127
Future prospect of EUS   16, 33, 132, 138

G

Gallbladder, normal   88
Gallbladder cancer   95, 117
Gallbladder disease   87–95

Gallbladder polyp   90, 98
Gallbladder wall   88
Gallstone   88, 98
Gastric cancer   60–67, 110, 146
Gastric neoplasm   109
Gastric wall, normal   9–14, 38, 45, 58, 59, 144, 145
Gastrointestinal wall   9–15, 38–40, 45

H

Hemangioma   123
Hamartoma, multiple biliary   125
Hepatocellular carcinoma   125
Hyperplasia, hepatic   127

I

Instrument   2, 29–32
Intestinal wall, echographic pattern of   15, 39, 40, 45

K

Klatskin tumor   117

L

Laparoscopic sonography   119–131
    method   121
Laparoscopic ultrasonography   *see* Laparoscopic sonography
Leiomyoblastoma, gastric   47, 110
Leiomyoma
    of esophagus   106, 143
    of stomach   46, 110, 146
Leiomyosarcoma   46, 69, 110
Liver, normal   153
Liver disease   119–131

M

Machida EPB-503BL   3
Malignant gastrointestinal disease   56–71
Malignant lymphoma   69, 111
Mechanical scanning   18, 19
Menétrier's disease   52
Metastatic lymph node   67
Multiple biliary hamartoma   125

N

Non-Hodgkin lymphoma   111

Normal gastrointestinal wall   9–15, 38, 39, 45, 57–59
    colonic wall   39, 60, 150
    duodenal wall   14, 39, 60, 148, 149
    esophageal wall   6–8, 57, 58, 141, 142
    gallbladder wall   88
    gastric wall   9–14, 38, 45, 58, 59, 144, 145
    rectal wall   39, 40, 150

O

Obliteration of main pancreatic duct   84
Olympus GF-UM2/EUM2   3
Olympus LPS-UM1/EUM1   119–121

P

Pancreas, normal   73, 155
Pancreatic cancer   72–78, 112, 156
    diagnostic efficiency   77
Pancreatic cyst   85
Pancreatic duct, dilatation of   83
    obliteration of   84
    stenosis of   84
Pancreatic examination   79
Pancreatic pseudocyst   112
Pancreatitis, chronic   76, 79–86
    pseudotumorous   84
Pancreatolith   82
Papilla cancer   67, 101
Papilla of Vater   101, 158
Papillitis   101
Periampullary tumor   114
Polyp, colonic   54
    gallbladder   90, 98
Prostate   151
Pseudocyst, pancreatic   112
Pseudotumorous pancreatitis   84

R

Radial scanning type   18, 19
Rectal cancer   152
Rectal wall, normal   39, 40, 150
Rectosigmoid cancer   152
Rectosigmoid colon   150
Resectability of GI tumors   106–118

S

Scanning way   4
Scanning technique   3–16
Sector scanning   19

Sigmoid colon, normal   150
Solitary tuberculoma   128
Sonolaparoscope   120
Sonolaparoscopy   120-122
Stenosis of main pancreatic duct   84
Submucosal tumor, gastric   46, 69, 147

T

Transducer   *see* Ultrasonic transducer
Tuberculoma, solitary   128

U

Ulcer, duodenal   50
    gastric   49, 50, 147, 148
Ulcerative colitis   53
Ultrasonic endoscope
    development   18-34
    electronic scanning   18, 19
    fundamental criteria   19
    history   18
    laparoscope   32
    linear scanning type   18, 19
    mechanical scanning   18, 19
    principle   26, 31
    prototype of gastrofiberscope   2, 20-32
    prototype for lower GI examination   33
    radial scanning type   18, 19
    scanning methods   18
    sector scanning   19
    trial model   *see* prototype
Ultrasonic transducer   1-4, 22, 27, 31
    transesophageal   1
    transrectal   1
    transurethral   1
Ultrasonographic examination of pancreas   79
Ultrasound interaction with GI wall   35-43
Uterus   151